Sports Spine

Editors

ADAM L. SHIMER
FRANCIS H. SHEN

CLINICS IN SPORTS MEDICINE

www.sportsmed.theclinics.com

Consulting Editor
MARK D. MILLER

July 2021 • Volume 40 • Number 3

ELSEVIER

1600 John F. Kennedy Boulevard • Suite 1800 • Philadelphia, Pennsylvania, 19103-2899

http://www.theclinics.com

CLINICS IN SPORTS MEDICINE Volume 40, Number 3
July 2021 ISSN 0278-5919, ISBN-13: 978-0-323-81389-1

Editor: Lauren Boyle
Developmental Editor: Diana Grace Ang

Clinics in Sports Medicine (ISSN 0278-5919) is published quarterly by Elsevier Inc., 360 Park Avenue South, New York, NY 10010-1710. Months of issue are January, April, July, and October. Business and Editorial Offices: 1600 John F. Kennedy Blvd., Ste. 1800, Philadelphia, PA 19103-2899. Customer Service Office: 3251 Riverport Lane, Maryland Heights, MO 63043. Periodicals postage paid at New York, NY and additional mailing offices. Subscription prices are $364.00 per year (US individuals), $931.00 per year (US institutions), $100.00 per year (US students), $405.00 per year (Canadian individuals), $964.00 per year (Canadian institutions), $100.00 (Canadian students), $475.00 per year (foreign individuals), $964.00 per year (foreign institutions), and $235.00 per year (foreign students). Foreign air speed delivery is included in all *Clinics* subscription prices. All prices are subject to change without notice. **POSTMASTER:** Send address changes to *Clinics in Sports Medicine*, Elsevier Health Sciences Division, Subscription Customer Service, 3251 Riverport Lane, Maryland Heights, MO 63043. Customer Service (orders, claims, online, change of address): Elsevier Health Sciences Division, Subscription Customer Service, 3251 Riverport Lane, Maryland Heights, MO 63043. **Tel: 1-800-654-2452 (U.S. and Canada); 314-447-8871 (outside U.S. and Canada). Fax: 314-447-8029. E-mail: journalscustomerservice-usa@elsevier.com (for print support); journalsonlinesupport-usa@elsevier.com (for online support).**

Reprints. For copies of 100 or more of articles in this publication, please contact the Commercial Reprints Department, Elsevier Inc., 360 Park Avenue South, New York, NY 10010-1710. Tel.: 212-633-3874; Fax: 212-633-3820; E-mail: reprints@elsevier.com.

Clinics in Sports Medicine is covered in *MEDLINE/PubMed (Index Medicus) Current Contents/Clinical Medicine, Excerpta Medica,* and *ISI/Biomed.*

Contributors

CONSULTING EDITOR

MARK D. MILLER, MD
S. Ward Casscells Professor, Department of Orthopaedics, University of Virginia, Consultant Team Physician, James Madison University Founder, Miller Review Course Vice President AOSSM, Harrisonburg, Virginia

EDITORS

ADAM L. SHIMER, MD
Associate Professor, Department of Orthopaedic Surgery, University of Virginia, Charlottesville, Virginia

FRANCIS H. SHEN, MD
Warren G. Stamp Endowed Professor, Professor of Pediatrics, Head of Orthopaedic Spine Division, Department of Orthopaedic Surgery, University of Virginia, Charlottesville, Virginia

AUTHORS

KEITH R. BACHMANN, MD
Assistant Professor, Department of Orthopaedic Surgery, University of Virginia, Charlottesville, Virginia

KEVEN S. BURNS, MD
Spine Institute of Arizona, Scottsdale, Arizona

CHRISTOPHER C. CHUNG, BS
Medical Student, Department of Orthopaedic Surgery, University of Virginia, Charlottesville, Virginia

EDWARD J. DOHRING, MD
Spine Institute of Arizona, Scottsdae, Arizona

CHELSEA D. FROST, MD, MS
Department of Orthopedics, Emory University, Atlanta, Georgia

GEORGE W. FRYHOFER, MD, MTR
Resident Physician, Department of Orthopaedic Surgery, University of Pennsylvania, Philadelphia, Pennsylvania

PAUL R. GAUSE, MD
Spine Institute of Arizona, Scottsdale, Arizona

JOSEPH P. GJOLAJ, MD
Associate Professor of Orthopaedic Surgery, Department of Orthopaedics, University of Miami Miller School of Medicine, Miami, Florida

RYAN J. GODINSKY, MD
Spine Institute of Arizona, Scottsdale, Arizona

HAMID HASSANZADEH, MD
Department of Orthopaedics, University of Virginia, Charlottesville, Virginia

DAVID HRYVNIAK, DO, CAQSM, RMSK
Assistant Professor, Department of Physical Medicine and Rehabilitation, University of Virginia, Charlottesville, Virginia

WELLINGTON K. HSU, MD
Clifford C. Raisbeck Distinguished Professor of Orthopaedic Surgery, Director of Research, Professor, Departments of Orthopaedic Surgery and Neurological Surgery, Northwestern University Feinberg School of Medicine, Chicago, Illinois

PRAMOD N. KAMALAPATHY, BA
Department of Orthopaedics, University of Virginia, Charlottesville, Virginia

MICHAEL MARKOWITZ, DO
Rowan University School of Osteopathic Medicine, Orthopedic Surgery, Stratford, New Jersey

ANDREW Z. MO, MD
Orthopaedic Spine Surgery Fellow, Department of Orthopaedics, University of Miami Miller School of Medicine, Miami, Florida

ADAM L. SHIMER, MD
Associate Professor, Department of Orthopaedic Surgery, University of Virginia, Charlottesville, Virginia

HARVEY E. SMITH, MD
Associate Professor, Department of Orthopaedic Surgery, University of Pennsylvania Perelman School of Medicine, Philadelphia, Pennsylvania

ROBERT G. WATKINS, III, MD
Co-Director, Marina Spine Center, Marina del Rey, California

ROBERT G. WATKINS, IV, MD
Co-Director, Marina Spine Center, Marina del Rey, California

BARRETT WOODS, MD
The Rothman Institute at Thomas Jefferson University Hospital, Philadelphia, Pennsylvania

Contents

history, physical examination, and diagnostic imaging are important to distinguish spondylolysis from other causes of lower back pain. Early pars stress reaction can be identified with advanced imaging, before the development of cortical fracture or vertebral slip progression to spondylolisthesis. Conservative management is first-line for low-grade injury with surgical intervention indicated for refractory symptoms, severe spondylolisthesis, or considerable neurologic deficit. Prompt diagnosis and management of spondylolysis leads to good outcomes and return to competition for most athletes.

Back pain in sport is a common complaint and seen by athletes, trainers, and treating physicians. Although there are a multitude of pain generators, mechanical sources are most common. Certain sports can lead to increased mechanical and axial loading, such as competitive weightlifting and football. Common mechanical causes of pain include disk herniation and spondylolysis. Patients typically respond to early identification and conservative treatment. In others, surgical intervention is required to provide stability and prevent long-term sequelae.

Lumbar disk herniation is the most common surgical condition of the spine. High-level athletes participate in activities that place extreme loads on the intervertebral disks. These repetitive loads may lead to an elevated risk for degenerative disk disease, which in turn predisposes to disk herniations. Treatment algorithms for athletes with disk herniations are similar to those in the nonathletic population; however, success in the athletic population is often measured in the ability to return to play. Both nonoperative and operative treatment show a high success rate in return to play in athletes treated for disk herniations.

The key to successful treatment of elite athletes is optimizing the medical care at every step: injury prevention and sport-specific training; comprehensive history and physical examination; high-quality and complete diagnostic studies; accurate diagnosis; control and completion of rehabilitation program; minimally invasive, safe, and effective surgeries; risk assessment for return to sport; guided and gradual return to sport; and continued rehabilitation and exercise program after return to sport.

Idiopathic scoliosis will be noted in 2% to 3% of typically developing athletes. Sports physicals are an opportunity to screen for spinal deformity and to promote healthy involvement in activities. Bracing is effective at limiting further progression especially if a curve progresses beyond 20°. If spinal fusion is performed, most surgeons allow return to noncontact and contact sports by 6 to 12 months. There are many other conditions associated with scoliosis that require a more nuanced approach and assessment of the entire patient. Patients with Down syndrome should be examined for myelopathy before participation and a lateral radiograph obtained if concerned for instability.

Although the safety of contact sports has improved over the years, participation in any sport always carries a risk of injury. When cervical or lumbar spine injuries do occur, prompt diagnosis is essential, and athletes must be held out of the sport if indicated to prevent further harm and allow for recovery. This article highlights some of the most common cervical spine pathologies (stinger/burners, strain, stenosis/cord neuropraxia, disc herniation, and fracture/instability) and lumbar spine pathologies (strain, disc degeneration, disc herniation, fracture, spondylolysis/spondylolisthesis, and scoliosis) encountered in sports and reviews the associated return to play guidelines and expectations for each condition.

Aging athletes face unique, increased adversities related to increased mobility and age-related spine issues, such as spinal stenosis, osteoporosis complicated by fragility fractures, and degenerative disk disease. This article covers various spine pathologies that aging athletes experience and ideal treatment of this population to allow safe return to activity.

CLINICS IN SPORTS MEDICINE

SERIES OF RELATED INTERESTED

Orthopedic Clinics
https://www.orthopedic.theclinics.com/
Foot and Ankle Clinics
https://www.foot.theclinics.com/
Hand Clinics
https://www.hand.theclinics.com/
Physical Medicine and Rehabilitation Clinics
https://www.pmr.theclinics.com/

THE CLINICS ARE AVAILABLE ONLINE!
Access your subscription at:
www.theclinics.com

Foreword

Sports Medicine Is not Spineless!

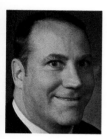

Mark D. Miller, MD
Consulting Editor

We try to be all-inclusive and comprehensive in our coverage of topics in *Clinics in Sports Medicine*. Although my practice does not include spine, spine is certainly a part of a sports medicine practice. At our institution, we are lucky to have not one but two "sports spine" specialists, each covering a Division I college that we care for— …and they both get a lot of referrals from those training rooms. These two surgeons, Drs Frank Shen and Adam Shimer, agreed to put together a treatise on the care of spine problems in athletes so that even if you don't actually practice sports spine, you will know when and how urgently to refer your athletes to the spine experts on your sports medicine team.

This issue is well organized and comprehensive. It begins with injury prevention and then focuses on on-field management. What follows is an overview of various spine conditions commonly seen in athletes. Young and old athletes alike are covered, and the important issue of Return to Play is addressed. My sincere thanks to Drs Shen and Shimer—now let's "get back to it."

Mark D. Miller, MD
Division of Sports Medicine
Department of Orthopaedic Surgery
University of Virginia
Charlottesville, VA, USA

Miller Review Course
Harrisonburg, VA, USA

513 Half Mile Branch Road
Crozet, VA 22932, USA

E-mail address:
MDM3P@hscmail.mcc.virginia.edu

Clin Sports Med 40 (2021) ix
https://doi.org/10.1016/j.csm.2021.04.005
0278-5919/21/© 2021 Published by Elsevier Inc.

Preface

Not Just Shoulders and Knees: An Athlete Has a Spine too!

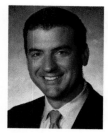 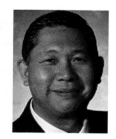

Adam L. Shimer, MD   Francis H. Shen, MD
Editors

Welcome to this issue of *Clinic in Sports Medicine* focused solely on the axial skeleton and its care in the athlete-patient. Although commonly overlooked in sports circles, spine-related injuries, pain, and limitations remain a commonly encountered complaint among the athletes that you care for. Furthermore, spine remains an area that most general orthopedists and sports medicine specialists are less than comfortable diagnosing and managing. We hope that this work will provide an athlete-focused framework from foundational basics to contemporary surgical techniques all written with the *Clinic in Sports Medicine* readership in mind. Like much of orthopedics, a huge component of spine care is education and prevention; this is particularly true in athletes, from weekend warrior to professional. Similar to a rotator cuff protocol or knee proprioception routine, we encourage a sports medicine specialist with team affiliation to consider introducing a core-strengthening and pelvic stabilization program to their system. We believe that with this training component they will see a decrease in the severity and number of spine issues. Even the most diligent preventative core program will not prevent all spine problems. If spine complaints do arise, thankfully the vast majority of them are self-limiting and resolve with thoughtful, diligent conservative care.

The first, most important care is determining whether something is severe (such as spinal cord injury or cauda equina syndrome) and demands urgent/emergent spine surgery evaluation or if it is less urgent and can be worked up over a longer time course. We hope that this issue will help the sports medicine practitioner be more confident with this determination. Even painful radiculopathy or spondylolisthesis is routinely successfully treated with nonoperative care, such as rest, physical therapy, oral anti-inflammatory medicine, and/or injections. If the spinal condition remains painful, limits athletic performance, or is associated with neurologic deficits, surgery may be required. Although not a guarantee, modern, less invasive surgical techniques (cervical decompressions and MIS lumbar discectomies) are getting athletes back in

Clin Sports Med 40 (2021) xi–xii
https://doi.org/10.1016/j.csm.2021.04.004
0278-5919/21/© 2021 Published by Elsevier Inc.   sportsmed.theclinics.com

action at a more predictable rate and in a shorter time than ever before. Some conditions (such a severe congenital cervical stenosis) may preclude some contact athletes from returning to their sport.

Spine care in the athlete-patient is very rewarding for the same reason as knee and shoulder care in the same group. They are a high functioning group focused on restoration of function and return to sport. Thank you again for taking the time to look through this issue, and we hope you find it engaging and educational.

Adam L. Shimer, MD
Department of Orthopaedic Surgery
University of Virginia School of Medicine
PO Box 800159
Charlottesville, VA 22903, USA

Francis H. Shen, MD
Department of Orthopaedic Surgery
University of Virginia School of Medicine
PO Box 800159
Charlottesville, VA 22903, USA

E-mail addresses:
shimer@virginia.edu (A.L. Shimer)
FHS2G@hscmail.mcc.virginia.edu (F.H. Shen)

Spine Injury Prevention

David Hryvniak, DO, CAQSM, RMSK[a,*], Chelsea D. Frost, MD, MS[b]

KEYWORDS

- Spinal injury • Kinesio taping • Spearing • Core stability • Cowboy collar

KEY POINTS

- Low back pain and spinal injury are a common pathology and disability among athletes that can be prevented.
- Core stability, flexibility, and Kinesio taping have been shown to be important adjuncts to any rehabilitation or spine injury prevention program.
- Equipment, technique, and rule changes are all important aspects of spine injury prevention in sports.

INTRODUCTION/INCIDENCE

Spinal injury or back pain is considered to be the leading cause of disability worldwide[1] and one of the most common symptoms for which patients seek medical care (**Table 1**). It is thought to have a lifetime incidence ranging between 60% and 90%, with 26% of people reporting an episode of low back pain within the previous 3 months.[2] The direct medical expenditures as well as the indirect costs through loss of work productivity and disability due to back pain are increasing, and in 2008 care related to back pain was estimated to be $86 billion.[3] Up to 25% of all workdays missed in the United States are attributed to low back pain,[4] and more than 75% of episodes have no clear diagnosis.[5] Among athletes, low back pain has been shown to have a lifetime prevalence ranging between 33% and 84% with variability based on one's sport participation. The highest prevalence of low back pain was noted in skiers, floorball players, and rowers, whereas the lowest prevalence was found in shooters, golfers, and triathletes.[6] Although most patients will have near-complete resolution of symptoms within 30 days of onset, some will have persistent pain lasting for more than 90 days. In addition, some patients may experience resolution of symptoms but also experience episodes of recurrent pain.

[a] Department of Physical Medicine & Rehabilitation, University of Virginia, 545 Ray C Hunt Drive, Charlottesville, VA 22908, USA; [b] Department of Orthopedics, Emory University, Atlanta, GA, USA
* Corresponding author.
E-mail address: Djh3f@virginia.edu

Clin Sports Med 40 (2021) 429–444
https://doi.org/10.1016/j.csm.2021.03.001
0278-5919/21/© 2021 Elsevier Inc. All rights reserved.

Table 1
Core exercises for the spine

Exercise Type	Muscle Group	Number of Repetitions	Number of Days per Week	Number of Weeks
Strengthening Exercises				
Plank	Back extensors, quadratus lumborum, erector spinae, abdominals	5–10	Daily	4–6
Side bridges[a]	Quadratus lumborum	10–20	Daily	4–6
Hip bridges	Back and hip extensors, gluteal muscles, hamstrings	10–20	Daily	4–6
Bird dog	Back extensors, erector spinae, gluteal muscles	10–20	Daily	4–6
Abdominal bracing	Abdominals	10–20	Daily	4–6
Stretching Exercises				
Cat back stretch	Middle and lower back	5–10	Daily	4–6
Kneeling back extension stretch	Low back	5–10	Daily	4–6
Seated side straddle	Adductors, medial hamstrings, semitendinosus, semimembranosus	5–10	Daily	4–6
Piriformis stretch	Piriformis, external and internal rotators	5–10	Daily	4–6
Knee to chest stretch	Quadratus lumborum	5–10	Daily	4–6

[a] Can perform modified side bridges.
- Heat should be applied to the lower back for 15 to 20 minutes before performing the exercises.
- Pain should not be experienced during exercises. If pain does worsen or it does not improve after performing exercises for 3 to 4 weeks, discuss with your physician.
- Exercises should be performed in conjunction with a progressive cardiovascular training program that consists of aerobic exercises (ie, walking, swimming, cycling) for 30 minutes, 3 to 5 days per week. When performing aerobic exercises, the spine should be maintained in neutral position while stabilizing the abdominal muscles.

CORE STABILITY STRENGTHENING/REHABILITATION

In recent years, core strengthening has become a major trend in rehabilitation and is a term used to describe the muscular control required around the lumbar spine to maintain functional stability. The "core" is described as a box with the abdominals in the front, paraspinals and gluteals in the back, the diaphragm as the root, and the pelvic floor and hip girdle musculature as the bottom.[7] It both functional and athletic events, the core provides proximal stability for distal mobility.[8] Trunk musculature helps to stabilize the core by compressing and stiffening the spine.[9] In addition, intraabdominal pressures increase as core muscular contracts,[10] further increasing spinal stiffness and subsequently enhancing core stability.[11]

However, there remains considerable debate regarding which core muscles are the most important in optimizing spinal stability, specifically regarding the importance of transversus abdominis and multifidi musculature.[9,12–14] In patients without lumbar pathology, the transversus abdominis muscle has been shown to contract before upper extremity motion irrespective of the direction of motion.[15] In contrast, there is a substantial delay in activation of the transversus abdominis in patients with lumbar pathology with all movements, indicating a motor control deficit that can result in inefficient spine stabilization.[16] A lack of sufficient coordination within the core musculature can lead to decreased efficiency of movements and compensatory patterns, thus leading to strain and overuse injuries.[17]

Although core strengthening can decrease the risk of injury by enhancing lumbar spine stability and has also been shown to decrease the risk of injury to lower extremities,[18,19] there is no strong relationship between core stability and performance,[20,21] and excessive spinal loading can also increase the risk of injury.[18] A study in 2002 reported that no single core muscle can be identified as the most important for lumbar spine stability, and furthermore, no single muscle contributed more than 30% to the overall spinal stability.[14] Therefore, lumbar spine stabilization exercises may be most effective when a focus is placed on relearning motor control of the entire spinal musculature under various loading conditions.[22]

A core exercise program is typically done in stages and with gradual progression. Initially the program will begin with restoration of normal muscle length and mobility with the goal of correcting any existing muscle imbalances to allow proper joint function and movement efficiency. Following this, activation of deep core musculature is taught via lumbopelvic stability exercises with eventual progression to incorporation of a physio ball. The final step involves transitioning to standing in order to facilitate function movement exercises that promote balance and coordination of precise movements.[17] When evaluating patients, it is important to also note that not all core exercises are appropriate for all individuals. Exercises that cause hip and trunk flexion can be problematic in those with lumbar disk pathologies due to increased intradiscal pressure and spinal compression[10,18] as well as those with osteoporosis due to the risk of vertebral compression fractures.[23] As such, these patients may benefit more from exercises that maintain a neutral spine and pelvis. Individuals with facet-mediated pain and vertebral or intervertebral foraminal stenosis may not tolerate lumbar extension–based exercises and may therefore better benefit from lumbar flexion–based exercises.[24]

One study[25] found that certain factors can be used to assess which patients will respond favorable to core stabilization exercises:

- Younger age (<40 years)
- Greater general flexibility (hamstring length > 90°, postpartum)
- Positive prone instability test
- Presence of aberrant movement during spinal range of motion (painful arc of motion, abnormal lumbopelvic rhythm, and using arms on thighs for support)

Another study[26] proposed certain physical modalities that can serve to predict a good response from stabilization exercises in postpartum women:

- Positive posterior pelvic pain provocation (P4) test (also referred to as "thigh thrust test")
- Positive active straight leg raise
- Positive pain provocation (persists greater than 5 sec after palpation) with palpation of posterior superior iliac spine region (long dorsal sacroiliac ligament)
- Positive pain provocation (persists great than 5 sec after palpation) with palpation of pubic symphysis
- Positive trendelenburg gait

Multiple studies[15,27–31] have demonstrated that there is a lack of proper core musculature recruitment and core weakness in patients with chronic low back and sacroiliac pain. There is also evidence of core musculature instability in high-level athletes, which can lead to additional musculoskeletal injuries.[8,32–34] These patients have been noted to have increased difficulty with balance and compensation for unexpected truncal perturbation. They have also been noted to have overactivation of superficial global musculature but impaired control and activation of deep spinal musculature.[17]

Although lumbar spine stabilization exercise programs have been effective in treating patients with chronic low back pain,[35] there has been no conclusive evidence to demonstrate that stabilization programs are more effective in treating patients with chronic low back pain as compared with a generalized, less-specific exercise program.[36] In addition, although there is some evidence that suggests core stabilization may help prevent injury in athletes,[32] these programs have not been well studied and have not been proved to enhance athletic performance.

Flexibility has been shown to assist patient with low back pain. Stretching muscles and fascia of the back, legs, and buttock such as the hamstrings, erector muscles of the spine, and hip flexors can help increase the range of motion of the spine and assist back pain.[37] Pilates and other flexibility exercises have been shown to decrease chronic low back pain.[38] Decreased flexibility in the hip flexors and lumbar extensors have been shown to increase lumbar lordosis, which can increase back pain.[39]

STRENGTHENING EXERCISES

Plank (**Fig. 1**):

- Patient should lie on their stomach with the forearms on the floor and elbows directly beneath the shoulders.
- As the abdominal muscles are tightened, lift the hips off the floor.
- As the gluteal muscles are squeezed, lift the knees off the floor.
- Keep the body straight and hold for 30 seconds. If unable to maintain this position, bring the knees back to the floor and hold with just the hips elevated.
- Slowly return to start position and rest for 30 seconds, then repeat.
- Throughout the exercise, do not let the pelvis sag toward the floor and keep the abdominals tight.
- Perform 5 to 10 repetitions per day for 4 to 6 weeks.

Side bridges (**Fig. 2**A) and modified version of side bridges (**Fig. 2**B):

- Patient lies on their side on the floor. Can be modified with knees bent at 90°.
- With the elbow bent 90°, patient contracts the abdominal muscles and lifts the hips off the floor as shown while keeping the body straight.

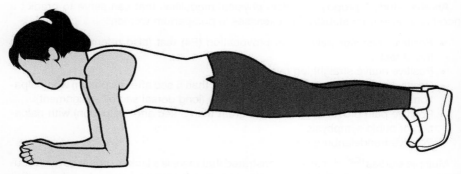

Fig. 1. Plank.

A

B

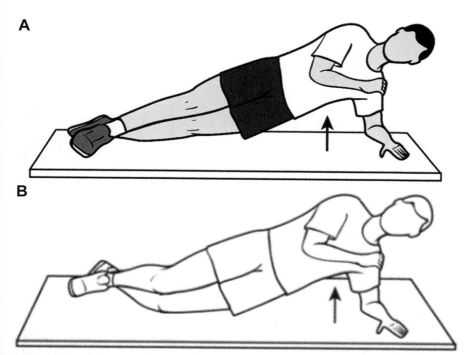

Fig. 2. (A) Side bridges. (B) Modified version of side bridges.

- Hold the position for 15 seconds then slowly return to neutral and repeat on the opposite side.
- Throughout the exercise, the patient should keep the neck in alignment with the spine and avoid shrugging the shoulders to the ear.
- Perform 10 to 20 repetitions per day on each side, for 4 to 6 weeks.

Hip bridges (**Fig. 3**):

- Patient lies on their back on the floor with arms either at the side or extended away from the body. Knees should be bend and feet flat on the floor.
- While contracting the abdominal and gluteal muscles, lift the pelvis up so that the body is in a straight line from the shoulders to knees.
- Hold this position for 10 seconds, then slowly lower the pelvis back to the floor.
- Throughout the exercise, keep the weight centered over the shoulder blades and do not tense up the neck muscles.
- Perform 10 to 20 repetitions per day for 4 to 6 weeks.

Bird dog (**Fig. 4**):

- Patient kneels on the floor on one's hands and knees. Hands should be about shoulder width apart.
- Lift the right arm straight out from the shoulder so that it is level with the body. At the same time, lift the left leg straight out from the hip.
- Hold this position for 5 to 10 seconds. One can gradually increase the hold time as tolerated while maintaining proper body position. Then slowly lower arm and leg back to neutral.
- Repeat with the opposite arm and leg.

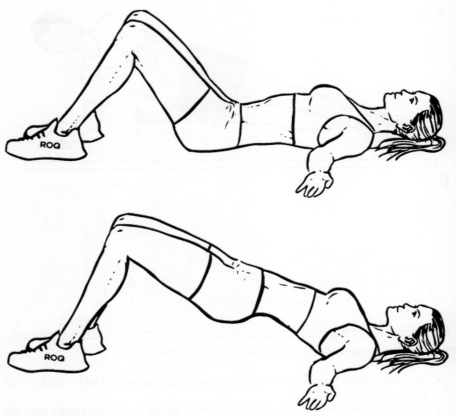

Fig. 3. Hip bridges.

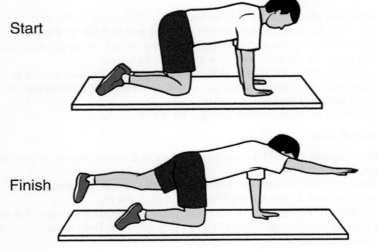

Start

Finish

Fig. 4. Bird dog.

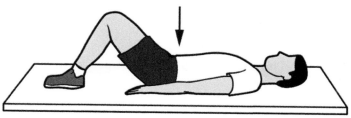

Fig. 5. Abdominal bracing.

- Throughout the exercise, keep the abdominal muscles tight and the back flat to stay balanced.
- Perform 10 to 20 repetitions per day on each side, for 4 to 6 weeks.

Abdominal bracing (**Fig. 5**):

- Patient lies on their back on the floor with arms at their sides. Knees should be bent and feet flat on the floor.
- Contract the abdominal muscles so that the stomach is pulled away from the waistband.
- Hold this position for 5 to 10 seconds.
- Throughout the exercise, keep the lower back flattened into the floor. It is important to not hold the breath and attempt to breathe normally.
- Perform 10 to 20 repetitions per day for 4 to 6 weeks.

STRETCHING EXERCISES

Cat back stretch (**Fig. 6**):

- Patient kneels on hands and knees in a relaxed position. Hands should be positioned directly under the shoulders.
- Raise the back up like a cat and hold for 30 seconds.
- Return to start position and relax for 30 seconds.

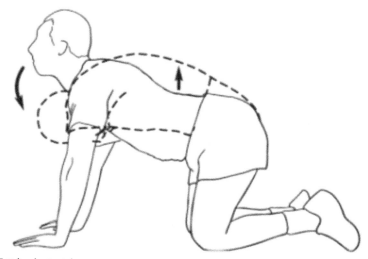

Fig. 6. Cat back stretch.

- Perform 5 to 10 repetitions per day for 4 to 6 weeks. Patients should feel the stretch in the lower back.

Kneeling back extension stretch (**Fig. 7**):

- Patient begins on hands and knees with hands positioned directly under the shoulders.
- Rock forward onto the arms while rounding the shoulders. Allow the lower back to drop toward the floor and hold this position for 5 seconds.
- Rock backward and sit the buttocks as close to heels as possible. Extend the arms and hold this position for 5 seconds.
- Throughout the exercise, look down toward the floor to keep the neck in neutral alignment with the spine.
- Perform 5 to 10 repetitions per day for 4 to 6 weeks. Patients should feel the stretch in the lower back and abdominals.

Seated side straddle (**Fig. 8**A) and modified version of seated side straddle (**Fig. 8**B):

- Patient sits on the floor with legs spread apart. If the patient is unable to tolerate sitting with both legs extended, it can be modified so that the patient sits on the floor with one leg extended to the side and the other leg bent as shown.
- Place both hands on the same ankle and bring the chin as close to the knee as possible. If patient is unable to grasp their ankle, can grasp the lower leg.
- Hold the maximum stretch for 30 seconds and then return to neutral and rest for 30 seconds.
- Repeat on the opposite site.

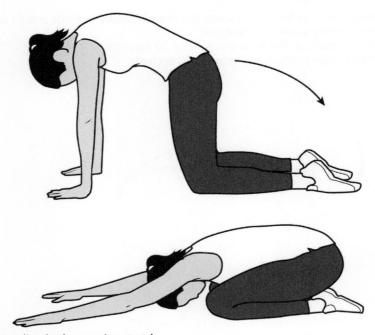

Fig. 7. Kneeling back extension stretch.

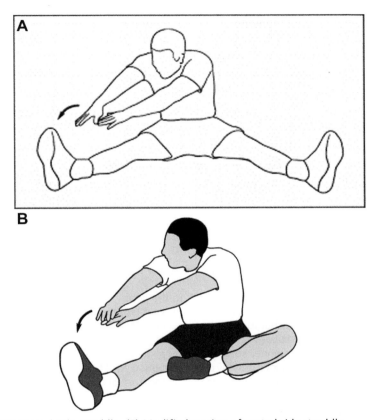

Fig. 8. (*A*) Seated side straddle. (*B*) Modified version of seated side straddle.

- Perform 5 to 10 repetitions per day on each side, for 4 to 6 weeks. Patient should feel this stretch in the hamstrings as well as the middle and lower back.

Piriformis stretch (**Fig. 9**):

- Patient should sit on the floor with both legs straight out in front, then one leg should be crossed over the other.
- Slowly twist toward the bent leg side, putting one hand behind for support. Place elbow of the opposite arm on the outside of the bent thigh and use to help twist further.
- Rotate the head and body in the direction of the supporting arm. Look over the shoulder and hold the stretch for 30 seconds.
- Slowly return to start position at center and rest for 30 seconds. Reverse positions and repeat on the opposite side.
- Perform 5 to 10 repetitions per day on each side, for 4 to 6 weeks. Patient should feel this stretch in the buttocks as well as at the sides.

Knee to chest stretch (**Fig. 10**):

- Patient lies on the floor with both legs extended.
- Lift one leg and bring knee toward the chest. While grasping the knee or shin, pull the leg in as far as it will go.

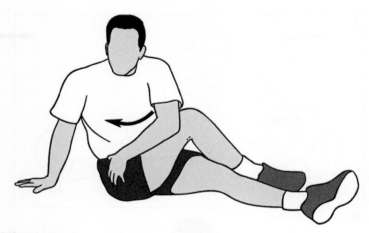

Fig. 9. Piriformis stretch.

- Tighten the abdominal muscles and press the spine into the floor. Hold this position for 5 seconds.
- Release the leg and slowly lower back to the floor.
- Repeat stretch on the other side with opposite leg, then return to start position.
- Pull both legs in together toward the chest and hold for 5 seconds before returning back to start position.
- Throughout the sequence, keep the spine aligned to the floor.
- Perform 5 to 10 repetitions per day of the sequence, for 4 to 6 weeks. Patient should feel this stretch in the lower back as well as the front of the hips and inner thigh.

KINESIO TAPING

Kinematic factors such as repeated or maximal loaded spinal flexion have been related to low back injury and pain.[40,41] In addition, lifting objects with high magnitudes of trunk flexion can increase the risk of developing low back pain[42] and has been identified as a risk factor for the development of occupation low back disorders.[43] In the 1970s Kinesio tape (KT), an elastic therapeutic tape, was developed by Dr Kenso Kase, and it has since been used for a variety of conditions including pain, swelling and edema, scar healing, proprioceptive facilitation, and musculature relaxation.[44,45] The appeal of its usage is the lack of need for ongoing time commitment or effort outside of the initial application and relatively inexpensive cost. The elastic capabilities of 120% to 140% of the initial length has been speculated to encourage or inhibit muscle mobility according to the muscle fiber direction.[45]

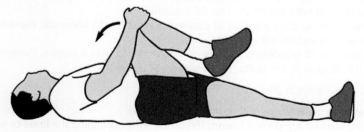

Fig. 10. Knee to chest stretch.

There have been multiple studies over the years evaluating the effectiveness of KT for low back pain, both as treatment and preventative methods; however, there has been no consensus on the benefit. These studies have evaluated both subjective and objective measures. Several studies have evaluated KT versus sham taping[46,47] with sham taping described simply as applying a strip of tape transversely immediately above the point of maximal pain. These have demonstrated insufficient evidence for the effect of KT on pain and disability, and subsequently limited evidence indicating that KT is superior to sham taping with respect to improving range of motion and muscular endurance. Furthermore, although one study[34] demonstrated significant improvement of endurance in the KT group at 1 week, there was no difference present at 8 weeks following conclusion of the intervention. In terms of studies evaluating use of KT alone or in conjunction with other therapies, it was demonstrated that KT, either as a sole treatment or in addition to another treatment, was no more effective in improving pain and disability outcomes when compared with other interventions.[48–50] One study[48] did indicate superiority of KT along with traditional physical therapy as compared with physical therapy alone at improving the movement-related cortical potential (MRCP). The MRCP is defined as the cerebral cortex activity extracted from electroencephalography in relation to voluntary movements. However, it should be mentioned that this study is considered to be a low-quality study in respect to the PEDro scale, which evaluates the validity and reliability of randomized controlled trials.[51–53]

The use and benefit of KT in terms of musculoskeletal injuries and pain have been evaluated by multiple studies. KT seems to have a small analgesic effect and may reduce disability, but there has been no clear evidence that KT is superior to other treatments. Furthermore, it is also unclear the clinical significance of these effects given in multiple studies has not demonstrated long-term benefit on follow-up. There has also been very little evidence demonstrating that KT, in combination with conventional physical therapy, is superior to physical therapy alone at improving motor control measures. There is a known association between pain and changes in motor control, range of motion, and muscular endurance. In the long term, these changes may lead to further tissue damage, lower pain threshold, altered posture, and encourage compensatory movement patterns.[54–56] It has therefore been speculated that KT improves proprioception by stimulating cutaneous mechanoreceptors, ultimately leading to increases in motor unit recruitment of the lumbar erector spinae muscles.[45]

Based on various studies, it can be inferred that although KT is not a substitute for other treatment modalities, it may be a useful supplement for management of spinal injuries and prevention and may allow better movement quality by improved range of motion and motor control. As reductions in pain have been demonstrated with sham taping, it was concluded that "KT applied with stretch to generate convolutions in the skin was no more effective than simple application of the tape without tension."[47] It was also shown that significant pain reductions were produced irrespective of tape placement or amount of stretch.[46,48–50] As such, it has been suggested that the precise method of taping may not be as critical to improving outcomes.

EQUIPMENT, TECHNIQUE, AND RULES FOR PREVENTION OF SPINE INJURY

Sport-related spine injury is a common problem in sports medicine. Approximately, 600,000 to 1.2 million football-related injuries occur in the United States annually; of these, between 10% and 25% involve the spine or axial skeleton.[57] Although contact sports often involve traumatic spine injuries, overuse spinal injuries are common in other sports such as gymnastics, dance, and soccer.

Equipment has been shown to have some effect on preventing spine injuries, especially in sports such as American football. Cowboy collars in football are often worn as part of equipment to prevent spinal injury. They have been shown to help decrease cervical hyperextension, which is often the mechanism for cervical spine injury in contact sports. They were not shown to prevent lateral neck flexion, which is common with brachial plexus traction injuries (ie, stingers, burners).[58]

Teaching proper tackling technique is an important factor in preventing spine injuries. The most common cause of this injury typically involves tackling with head-down contact and with the neck flexed, which can lead to axial loading. Head-down contact, defined as initiating contact with the top or crown of the helmet, is the only technique that results in axial loading. A recent CDC analysis showed head-first/head-down contact to be the cause of 8 of 28 deaths in HS and college football from 2005 to 2014.[59] The recommended tackling technique is to initiate contact with the chest or shoulder while keeping the head up. Heads-up tackling, in combination with an inside shoulder technique, provides a safer more effective technique.[60,61]

Technique, coaching, and preventative strength and conditioning are also an important consideration in other sports involving repetitive hyperextension and axial loading of the spine, and participation in these sports predisposes young athletes to pars fractures or spondylolysis. Common examples include baseball, gymnastics, football, tennis, and weight-lifting.[62]

Over the last several decades there has been an increased focus on preventing head and neck injuries that occur during sporting events. Given this raised awareness, there has been an effort to update and change the rules of the game to help decrease some of the circumstances that lead to these injuries. Starting in 1976 with Dr Torg, a thorough investigation of football-related spine injuries was undertaken. Dr Torq identified axial loading as a key aspect leading to spine injuries, often related to spearing.[63] Spearing is defined as a player lowering their head and using the crown of their helmet to initiate contact. Therefore, in 1976, a rule was instituted that made spearing illegal and even grounds of ejection, leading to a dramatic decrease in spinal injuries and quadriplegia.[64] More recently, there has been rule changes including shortening run backs on kickoffs, protecting defenseless players, and making any contact with the helmet illegal to decrease the risk of head and spinal injury.[65]

SUMMARY

Spinal injury prevention is a key aspect of the sports medicine care of an athlete, which can involve a strength and conditioning program, rehabilitation, equipment, mechanics/technique, as well as rule changes. These are all critical pieces that prevent spinal injury that can have a large effect on performance with a goal of preventing significant morbidity and disability.

CLINICS CARE POINTS

- Core stability and flexibility can be a helpful tool for both prevention and treatment of low back pain in athletes.

- Kinesio taping is not a substitute for other treatment modalities; however, it can be a useful supplement for management of spinal injuries and prevention and may allow better movement quality by improved range of motion and improved motor control.

- Heads-up tackling and rule changes regarding spearing have been critical for prevention of spinal injury.

DISCLOSURE

The authors have nothing to disclose.

REFERENCES

1. Hoy D, March L, Brooks P, et al. The global burden of low back pain: estimates from the global burden of disease 2010 study. Ann Rheum Dis 2014;73:968–74.
2. Deyo RA, Mirza SK, Martin BI. Back pain prevalence and visit rates: estimates from U.S. national surveys, 2002. Spine (Phila Pa 1976) 2006;31(23):2724–7.
3. American Academy of Orthopaedic Surgeons, Armstrong A, Hubbard MC. Overview of the spine. In: American Academy of Orthopaedic Surgeons, Armstrong A, Hubbard MC, editors. Essentials of musculoskeletal care. 5th edition. Jones & Bartlett Learning; 2018.
4. Devereaux M. Low back pain. Med Clin North Am 2009;93(2):477–x.
5. Bhatia NN, Chow G, Timon SJ, et al. Diagnostic modalities for the evaluation of pediatric back pain: a prospective study. J Pediatr Orthop 2008;28(2):230–3.
6. Farahbakhsh F, Rostami M, Noormohammadpour P, et al. Prevalence of low back pain among athletes: a systematic review. J Back Musculoskelet Rehabil 2018; 31(5):901–16.
7. Richardson C, Jull G, Hodges P, et al. Therapeutic exercise for spinal segmental stabilization in low back pain: scientific basis and clinical approach. Edinburg, NY: Churchill Livingstone; 1999.
8. Kibler WB, Press J, Sciascia A. The role of core stability in athletic function. Sports Med 2006;36(3):189–98.
9. McGill SM. Low back stability: from formal description to issues for performance and rehabilitation. Exerc Sport Sci Rev 2001;29(1):26–31.
10. Nachemson AL. Disc pressure measurements. Spine (Phila Pa 1976) 1981; 6(1):93–7.
11. Essendrop M, Andersen TB, Schibye B. Increase in spinal stability obtained at levels of intra-abdominal pressure and back muscle activity realistic to work situations. Appl Ergon 2002;33(5):471–6.
12. Hodges PW. Is there a role for transversus abdominis in lumbo-pelvic stability? Man Ther 1999;4(2):74–86.
13. Wilke HJ, Wolf S, Claes LE, et al. Stability increase of the lumbar spine with different muscle groups. A biomechanical in vitro study. Spine (Phila Pa 1976).20(2):192-198.
14. Morris SL, Lay B, Allison GT. Corset hypothesis rebutted–transversus abdominis does not co-contract in unison prior to rapid arm movements. Clin Biomech (Bristol, Avon) 2012;27(3):249–54.
15. Hodges PW, Richardson CA. Inefficient muscular stabilization of the lumbar spine associated with low back pain. A motor control evaluation of transversus abdominis. Spine (Phila Pa 1976) 1996;21(22):2640–50.
16. Teyhen DS, Miltenberger CE, Deiters HM, et al. The use of ultrasound imaging of the abdominal drawing-in maneuver in subjects with low back pain. J Orthop Sports Phys Ther 2005;35(6):346–55.
17. Akuthota V, Ferreiro A, Moore T, et al. Core stability exercise principles. Curr Sports Med Rep 2008;7(1):39–44.
18. Axler CT, McGill SM. Low back loads over a variety of abdominal exercises: searching for the safest abdominal challenge. Med Sci Sports Exerc 1997; 29(6):804–11.

19. Willson JD, Dougherty CP, Ireland ML, et al. Core stability and its relationship to lower extremity function and injury. J Am Acad Orthop Surg 2005;13(5):316–25.
20. Okada T, Huxel KC, Nesser TW. Relationship between core stability, functional movement, and performance. J Strength Cond Res 2011;25(1):252–61.
21. Reed CA, Ford KR, Myer GD, et al. The effects of isolated and integrated 'core stability' training on athletic performance measures: a systematic review. Sports Med 2012;42(8):697–706.
22. Cholewicki J, VanVliet JJ 4th. Relative contribution of trunk muscles to the stability of the lumbar spine during isometric exertions. Clin Biomech (Bristol, Avon) 2002; 17(2):99–105.
23. Sinaki M. Exercise for patients with osteoporosis: management of vertebral compression fractures and trunk strengthening for fall prevention. PM R 2012; 4(11):882–8.
24. Escamilla RF. Core stabilization. In: Miller MD, editor. Orthopaedic knowledge update: sports medicine 5. 5th edition. Walters Kluwer; 2018.
25. Hicks GE, Fritz JM, Delitto A, et al. Preliminary development of a clinical prediction rule for determining which patients with low back pain will respond to a stabilization exercise program. Arch Phys Med Rehabil 2005;86(9):1753–62.
26. Stuge B, Laerum E, Kirkesola G, et al. The efficacy of a treatment program focusing on specific stabilizing exercises for pelvic girdle pain after pregnancy: a randomized controlled trial. Spine (Phila Pa 1976) 2004;29(4):351–9.
27. Hodges PW. Core stability exercise in chronic low back pain. Orthop Clin North Am 2003;34:245Y254.
28. Hides JA, Richardson CA, Jull GA. Multifidusmuscle recovery is not automatic after resolution of acute, first-episode low back pain. Spine 1996;21:2763Y2769.
29. Arokoski JP, Valta T, Kankaanpää M, et al. Activation of lumbar paraspinal and abdominal muscles during therapeutic exercises in chronic low back pain patients. Arch Phys Med Rehabil 2004;85(5):823–32.
30. Newcomer KL, Jacobson TD, Gabriel DA, et al. Muscle activation patterns in subjects with and without low back pain. Arch Phys Med Rehabil 2002;83:816Y821.
31. Hungerford B, Gilleard W, Hodges P. Evidence of altered lumbopelvic muscle recruitment in the presence of sacroiliac joint pain. Spine 2003;28:1593Y1600.
32. Leeton DT, Ireland ML, Willson JD. Core stability measures as risk factors for lower extremity injury in athletes. Med Sci Sports Exerc 2004;36:926Y934.
33. Hewett TE, Lindenfeld TN, Riccobene JV, et al. The effect of neuromuscular training on the incidence of knee injury in female athletes. A prospective study. Am J Sports Med 1999;27:699Y706.
34. Heidt RS Jr, Sweeterman LM, Carlonas RL. Avoidance of soccer injuries with pre-season conditioning. Am J Sports Med 1999;27:699Y706.
35. Wang XQ, Zheng JJ, Yu ZW, et al. A meta-analysis of core stability exercise versus general exercise for chronic low back pain. PLoS One 2012;7(12):e52082.
36. Standaert CJ, Weinstein SM, Rumpeltes J. Evidence-informed management of chronic low back pain with lumbar stabilization exercises. Spine J 2008;8(1): 114–20.
37. MacAuley D, Best T. Evidence-based sports medicine. 2nd edition. Oxford, UK: Blackwell Publishing; 2007.
38. Gladwell V, Head S, Haggar M, et al. Does a program of pilates improve chronic non-specific low back pain? J Sport Rehabil 2006;15:338–50.
39. Nourbakhsh MR, Arabloo AM, Salavati M. The relationship between pelvic cross syndrome and chronic low back pain. J Back Musculoskelet Rehabil 2006;19: 119–28.

40. Adams MA, Hutton WC. Gradual disc prolapse. Spine (Phila Pa 1976) 1985;10(6): 524–31.

41. Hoogendoorn WE, Bongers PM, de Vet HC, et al. Flexion and rotation of the trunk and lifting at work are risk factors for low back pain: results of a prospective cohort study. Spine (Phila Pa 1976) 2000;25(23):3087–92.

42. Binh P, Ngo T, Amin Y, et al. Lifting height as the dominant risk factor for low-back pain and loading during manual materials handling: a scoping review. IISE Trans Occup Ergon Hum Factors 2017;5(3–4):158–71.

43. Fathallah FA, Marras WS, Parnianpour M. The role of complex, simultaneous trunk motions in the risk of occupation-related low back disorders. Spine (Phila Pa 1976) 1998;23(9):1035–42.

44. Mostafavifar M, Wertz J, Borchers J. A systematic review of the effectiveness of kinesio taping for musculoskeletal injury. Phys Sportsmed 2012;40(4):33–40.

45. Kase K, Kase T, Wallis J. Clinical therapeutic applications of the kinesio taping method. 2nd edition. Ken Ikai, Tokyo: Kinesio Taping Assoc; 2003.

46. Castro-Sánchez AM, Lara-Palomo IC, Matarán-Peñarrocha GA, et al. Kinesio Taping reduces disability and pain slightly in chronic non-specific low back pain: a randomised trial [published correction appears in J Physiother. 2012;58(3):143]. J Physiother 2012;58(2):89–95.

47. Parreira Pdo C, Costa Lda C, Takahashi R, et al. Kinesio taping to generate skin convolutions is not better than sham taping for people with chronic non-specific low back pain: a randomised trial. J Physiother 2014;60(2):90–6.

48. Bae SH, Lee JH, Oh KA, et al. The effects of kinesio taping on potential in chronic low back pain patients anticipatory postural control and cerebral cortex. J Phys Ther Sci 2013;25(11):1367–71.

49. Kachanathu SJ, Alenazi AM, Seif HE, et al. Comparison between Kinesio Taping and a traditional physical therapy program in treatment of nonspecific low back pain. J Phys Ther Sci 2014;26(8):1185–8.

50. Paoloni M, Bernetti A, Fratocchi G, et al. Kinesio Taping applied to lumbar muscles influences clinical and electromyographic characteristics in chronic low back pain patients. Eur J Phys Rehabil Med 2011;47(2):237–44.

51. Sherrington C, Herbert RD, Maher CG, et al. A database of randomized trials and systematic reviews in physiotherapy. Man Ther 2000;5(4):223–6.

52. Macedo LG, Elkins MR, Maher CG, et al. There was evidence of convergent and construct validity of Physiotherapy Evidence Database quality scale for physiotherapy trials. J Clin Epidemiol 2010;63(8):920–5.

53. Maher CG, Sherrington C, Herbert RD, et al. Reliability of the PEDro scale for rating quality of randomized controlled trials. Phys Ther 2003;83(8):713–21.

54. Cholewicki J, Greene HS, Polzhofer GK, et al. Neuromuscular function in athletes following recovery from a recent acute low back injury. J Orthop Sports Phys Ther 2002;32(11):568–75.

55. Radebold A, Cholewicki J, Polzhofer GK, et al. Impaired postural control of the lumbar spine is associated with delayed muscle response times in patients with chronic idiopathic low back pain. Spine (Phila Pa 1976) 2001;26(7):724–30.

56. Sipko T, Kuczyński M. Intensity of chronic pain modifies postural control in low back patients. Eur J Pain 2013;17(4):612–20.

57. Patel SA, Vaccaro AR, Rihn JA. Epidemiology of spinal injuries in sports. Oper Tech Sports Med 2013;21(3):146–51.

58. Gorden JA, Straub SJ, Swanik CB, et al. Effects of football collars on cervical hyperextension and lateral flexion. J Athl Train 2003;38(3):209–15.

59. Kucera KL, Yau RK, Register-Mihalik J, et al. Traumatic brain and spinal cord fatalities among high school and college football players—United States 2005-2014. MMWR Morb Mortal Wkly Rep 2017;65:1465–9.
60. Heck JF, Clarke KS, Peterson TR, et al. National Athletic Trainers' Association position statement: head-down contact and spearing in tackle football. J Athl Train 2004;39(1):101–11.
61. Stockwell DW, Blalock R, Podell K, et al. At-risk tackling techniques in American Football. Orthop J Sports Med 2020. https://doi.org/10.1177/2325967120902714.
62. Watkins RG. Lumbar spondylolysis and spondylolisthesis in athletes. Semin Spine Surg 2010;22(4):210–7.
63. Torg JS. Epidemiology,pathomechanics, and prevention of athletic iniuries to the cervical Spine. Med Sci Sports Exerc 1985;17:295–330.
64. Torg JS. Epidemiology,pathomechanics, and prevention of football induced cervical spine cord trauma. Exerc Spgll Sci Rev 1992;20:321–33.
65. National football league rule changes. Available at: https://operations.nfl.com/football-ops/nfl-ops-honoring-the-game/health-safety-rules-changes/. Accessed August 20, 2020.

On-Field Management of Suspected Spinal Cord Injury

Michael Markowitz, DO[a], Barrett Woods, MD[b],*

KEYWORDS

• On-field management • Acute spinal cord injury • Athlete specific considerations

KEY POINTS

- The success of on-field management of suspected spinal cord injury begins before the athlete steps onto the field through effective pregame planning among all medical staff.
- Medical staff should be well trained in all aspects of the athlete's care and one team leader should be predetermined to manage any suspected injury.
- Proper immobilization and equipment removal is essential and performed when necessary.

INTRODUCTION

Injury to the spine during sporting activities is a rare occurrence that ultimately demands a well-planned and multifaceted approach. These injuries can occur over a wide range of severity, from muscle strains and contusions, fractures, and dislocations, to even catastrophic spine injuries. A catastrophic spine injury is defined as an injury that causes structural distortion of the spinal column associated with the potential for, or actual, spinal cord injury (SCI).[1] Although these injuries affect athletes of all ages, preparation and planning begins before the athlete ever steps out onto the field.

Sport-related injury is the fourth most common cause of SCI (following motor vehicle accidents, falls, and acts of violence) and accounts for approximately 7.8% of injuries since 2015.[2] These traumas are devastating to an athlete and may lead to potentially permanent neurologic compromise or even a fatal outcome. Unlike typical trauma patients, athletes are often wearing helmets and other protective gear, especially in collision sports, which may complicate management of suspected spine injury. Although advances in sporting equipment have helped minimize SCI significantly, these injuries may still occur, demanding proper and expedient care so

The article submitted does not contain information pertaining to devices or drug names. No funds were received in support of this work. No disclosures.
[a] Rowan University School of Osteopathic Medicine Orthopedic Surgery, Stratford, NJ, USA;
[b] The Rothman Institute at Thomas Jefferson University Hospital, Philadelphia, PA, USA
* Corresponding author. Rothman Orthopaedics, 243 Hurffville - Cross Keys Road, Sewell, NJ 08080.
E-mail address: Barrett.Woods@rothmanortho.com

Clin Sports Med 40 (2021) 445–462
https://doi.org/10.1016/j.csm.2021.03.002
0278-5919/21/© 2021 Elsevier Inc. All rights reserved.

preparation is paramount. Well-trained medical staff should be present at each sporting event and assigned specific jobs to, not only be vigilant to injury on the field, but also have the skills necessary to evaluate, diagnose, and perform life-saving procedures. In addition, they should be well trained in equipment management and have knowledge of local hospitals capable of handling athletes with such injuries.

It is important for coaches to reinforce safety through practice of proper technique relevant to each sport. This can help minimize high-risk behavior during recreational and competitive play. Ultimately, understanding the epidemiology and mechanisms of SCI is essential to their prevention. The aim of this article was to review the on-field management of SCI from pregame preparation, mechanisms and types of injuries, on-field goals, and ultimately the escalation of an athlete's care.

EPIDEMIOLOGY

In athletics, there are nearly 12,000 spinal cord injuries each year, which primarily account for the second leading cause of SCI in the first 3 decades of life.[3,4] The cervical spine is most commonly injured, typically as a result of axial loading and flexion of the neck.[5] Less commonly, injury to the thoracolumbar spine can occur but is usually related to sport-specific degenerative processes.[3,6] High-risk sports include American football, hockey, rugby, skiing/snowboarding, and equestrian, with hockey accounting for the greatest number of catastrophic spine injuries overall.[7–9]

American football has gained a lot of attention when considering SCI in athletes. Although accounting for approximately 1% of these injuries, it is responsible for the highest incidence of SCI in the United States and remains under critical review due to the growing number of annual participants at all levels of play.[10] The patterns of spine injury in American football have evolved significantly over time, peaking in the 1960s with introduction of improved helmet design. Athletes were allowed to tackle head first (spear tackling) with the neck in slight flexion making contact with the crown of their head and their opponent. This places significant compressive axial forces through the cervical spine, predisposing the individual to spinal column and cord injury. Between 1971 and 1975, the National Football Head and Neck Injury Registry recorded 259 cases of unstable spine injuries and 99 cases of quadriplegia that were attributed to this aggressive, head-first, tackling.[11] As this danger was recognized, in January of 1976, head-first tackling was banned from high school, collegiate, and National Football Leagues (NFL) and over the following 10 years a 70% decrease in cervical spine injury and quadriplegia was reported.[12]

Similarly, the National Hockey League (NHL) responded to the prevalence of SCI through implementing league rule changes as well. Reports from Canada demonstrated 311 SCIs, 82.8% cervical injuries, in hockey between 1943 and 2005.[8] Many of these injuries were provoked from skating into the boards or being checked from behind. Since 2001, these injuries have substantially decreased as a result of rule modifications now preventing illegal checking. Athletes are now prohibited from checking another athlete from behind, as head-first contact into the board or onto the ice in a forward and flexed position significantly increases their risk of sustaining an SCI.[7,9] This was later followed in 2010 by the NHL prohibiting lateral or blind-sided checks to the patient's head and US Hockey raising the age of legal checking from 12 to 14 to minimize injury.[3] Similar to the NFL and NHL, all sports leagues should regularly review and implement rules to improve in-game safety and protection of the athletes.

Congenital anomalies of the spine can also predispose an athlete to SCI on the field. Although such anomalies pose unique challenges to medical professionals due to the lack of unified guidelines, the safety of these athletes in contact sports is unclear. Cervical stenosis has been identified as an important factor in the occurrence of neurologic injury following spine trauma, particularly due to a decreased sagittal canal diameter.[13,14] Torg and colleagues[15] defined a ratio on radiographic imaging to look at the anterior to posterior diameter of the spinal canal in comparison with the vertebral body and found that the ratio of less than 0.80 predisposed football players to transient neurologic injury. However, this ratio was later found to have a low positive predictive value based on statistical analysis and was not recommended for use in screening athletes.

Aebli and colleagues[16] used MRI to study athletes with SCI and reported that those with such injuries had overall smaller spinal canal diameter. They found that a midsagittal intervertebral disk space diameter of 8 mm was the best measurement and most predictive of SCI after cervical trauma. Overall, studies have shown that even with canal narrowing in high-contact athletes, the incidence of neurologic involvement is relatively small and should not be an absolute contraindication to athletic participation.[17,18] However, a discussion should be had between athletes and medical providers after one experiences a neurologic injury in conjunction with a congenital abnormality, and they should reconsider further participation in contact sports.

ON-FIELD INJURIES TO THE SPINE

There are a wide range of on-field injuries to the spine, and observation and diagnosis are key in the immediate moments after an injury. Although some injuries may require only a short period of rest, most may elicit a permanent injury if not appropriately handled. Therefore, trained medical staff should be cognizant of the mechanism of injury and clinical presentations that follow to properly handle the injured athlete on the field. Injuries range from transient neuropraxias, acute disk herniations, to fractures and dislocations; regardless, if neurologic symptoms present, especially involving bilateral extremities, extreme care in management should be performed.

STINGERS/BURNERS

Collision athletes who develop acute neurologic symptoms limited to one upper extremity may be considered to have a transient neuropraxia. These are very common injuries, also known as stingers or burners, that occur in many sports including American football, rugby, hockey, gymnastics, boxing, and weight lifting.[19] In particular, stingers have been reported in as many as 65% of college football players within their careers and in as many as one-third of all rugby players within a single season.[20] Typically this injury occurs as a result of 1 of 3 mechanisms: (1) a traction injury to the brachial plexus as a result of forced contralateral neck sidebending and ipsilateral depression of the shoulder; (2) direct compression to Erb's point of the brachial plexus; (3) cervical nerve root compression in the neural foramen after extreme extension and sidebending.[18,21,22] Athletes experiencing a stinger will complain of burning pain in the involved extremity with transient motor and sensory deficits in a nondermatomal pattern most commonly affecting the C5-6 nerve roots.

Stingers can last from seconds to hours after insult but usually resolve without intervention. Many times athletes will have complete resolution of symptoms and can be cleared to play when full range of motion and motor strength have occurred.[23] If symptoms persist, the athlete should not be cleared to play. In addition, if any concern for worsening symptoms of neck pain, weakness, involvement of the lower extremity, or clinical suspicion of a catastrophic spine injury, the athlete should be taken to the nearest SCI or trauma center for imaging and frequent neurologic monitoring.[24]

ACUTE DISK HERNIATION

Intervertebral disk herniations are a common cause of neck and back pain. These injuries occur commonly in contact athletes, more so than in the general populations, secondary to repetitive stresses athletes place on their spine, predisposing them to early degenerative processes.[25] From this, injury to the annulus fibrosus allows for herniation of the nucleus pulposus into the spinal canal causing compression on the nerves or spinal cord creating an array of symptoms from transient to permanent neurologic deficits. In high-contact sports, these stresses predispose athletes to cervical disk herniations commonly seen in the C3-4 and C5-6 levels.[26] Particularly in football (lineman and defensive backs) or rugby (front row forwards) there is an especially high incidence of cervical disk herniation due to the mechanics and repetition of their play.[27] In addition, athletes may suffer similar injury to the lower back, where herniations are commonly seen at L4-5 and L5-S1 levels, accounting for 90% of symptomatic cases.[28] Particularly, in football, lineman were found to be at an increased risk of acute disk herniation due to the a culmination of factors such as their training regimen, body weight, and repeated spine hyperextension during play.[27]

On the field, initial neurologic symptoms should prompt emergent immobilization during the primary survey and ultimately escalation of care to ensure any neurologic deficits can be minimized or handled when necessary.

FRACTURES AND DISLOCATIONS

Fractures to the cervical spine most commonly occur in the subaxial spine with injury patterns predicated on the mechanism of injury. The response to the spine and surrounding soft tissues is dependent on the neck position at the time of impact and can lead to a wide range of injury severity. When the cervical spine is in neutral alignment, the natural lordosis allows the energy of a collision to be distributed throughout the surrounding musculature and ligaments. However, when the spine is in an exaggerated flexion or extension position, reducing the innate lordotic alignment, compressive forces place higher stresses on the bony support predisposing to fractures and dislocations.[29]

Hyperflexion injuries are the most commonly reported neck injuries sustained by athletes.[30] Mechanistically, the cervical spine experiences an axial load while in some degree of flexion, thereby causing compression to the anterior column while the posterior elements experience tension forces creating a "tear-drop" fragment. Although these injuries involve varying degrees of posterior column involvement, they are inherently unstable, and range from posterior ligamentous injury to bilateral facet dislocations.[31,32]

The second most common injury experienced by athletes is a compressive burst fracture. These injuries occur after a pure axial compression to a neutrally aligned spine, which creates a rise in the intradiskal pressure resulting in failure of both the anterior and middle columns of the vertebral body.[29] If the injury is severe enough, SCI can occur secondary to retropulsion of bony fragments into the spinal canal. Burst fractures can also, and most commonly occur, without neurologic compromise, but this does not preclude immediate spinal stabilization. Again, the severity and ultimate treatment will be dictated by the integrity of the posterior ligamentous complex.

Hyperextension injuries to the spine are rare but result in significant injury. Athletes experiencing a large posterior force to the head will experience failure of the anterior longitudinal ligament and annulus fibrosus.[33] When these injuries are severe, there can be enough force to cause failure of the posterior ligamentous complex leading to posterior translation of the vertebral body into the spinal canal resulting in SCI.[34]

SCI to the upper cervical spine from fractures and dislocations are also rare. Although high-level injury can render a patient reliant on mechanical ventilation indefinitely, oftentimes these injuries do not elicit neurologic compromise. This is twofold, (1) because the space available for the cord at the upper cervical levels is greater than at the subaxial levels, and (2) because the common fracture patterns of the atlas (Jefferson fracture) and axis (traumatic spondylolisthesis), actually expand the diameter available for the spinal cord when they occur.[29] However, injuries of concern include those that render the atlanto-axial joint unstable, transverse ligament injury, and variants of odontoid fractures.

Ultimately, any suspicion of an SCI, whether through observation of the injury or through clinical examination demonstrating neurologic deficits, prompt immobilization and escalation of care are warranted.

THORACOLUMBAR INJURIES

Thoracolumbar spine injuries commonly result in benign muscle strains and contusions that respond well to nonoperative management, but these injuries can exist over a wide range including ligamentous instability and fractures.[7] This is because of the innate stability of the thoracolumbar spine is secondary to its surrounding structural support.[35] Injury develops when the extrinsic forces overpower the intrinsic stability of these supporting structures, creating potential for catastrophic injury and neurologic compromise.[3,6]

Particular injury patterns are often sport-specific, although football and hockey have the highest association with more severe damage to the spine's structural support; other sports such as in skiing and snowboarding place athletes at a high risk for catastrophic spine injury as well. Gymnasts on the other hand, experience injury through repetitive flexion-extension forces to the posterior elements and can thereby develop stress fractures to the pars interarticularis.[7] Ultimately, traumatic injuries are less commonly seen in these areas of the spine, and are typically related to degeneration from sport-specific activity leading to disk degeneration, herniation, spondylolysis, and others. Regardless of the type of injury, whether cervical or thoracolumbar, management of a suspected SCI should be focused on safe and urgent immobilization and escalation to a higher level of care (this management is discussed in a later section).

PREPARING FOR THE GAME

Before athletes step onto the field, sporting facilities, medical personnel, coaches, and nearby hospitals should collaborate to create protocols designed to effectively manage injured athletes with suspected SCI. First, knowledge of the sporting facility is paramount, all staff should understand routes into and out of sporting facilities to allow timely entrance and departure of emergency medical services (EMS). Although oftentimes the athlete may require up to 6 to 8 people to secure and stabilize a suspected spine injury, it is essential that effective communication occurs.[3] To accomplish this, a lead medical provider should be assigned to run all situations, this individual's goal is to predesignate jobs to the support staff through organized instructions while EMS is on the way. This job not only spans the time of injury but during pregame preparation, ensuring all appropriate materials are well stocked and easily accessible (eg, backboards, cervical collars, screw drivers, airway management and life support kits, automated external defibrillators [AEDs]), in addition to all ancillary staff being appropriately trained in the use of these tools and equipment management. In emergent situations, the patient may not always be able to communicate to the lead medical provider, so readily available and updated emergency contact information is essential before each event; it may even benefit all parties if families are introduced to the medical staff members at the beginning of each season which may help ease the anxiety in a dire situation.[6]

Ultimately, a suspected catastrophic spine injury will require an escalation of care from the field to a center capable of treating SCIs. Studies have shown that significant neurologic improvement was seen in athletes with SCI when transported directly to these specialty centers rather than to the nearest hospital.[36] Knowledge of such facilities should be predetermined before each game to avoid delay in the athlete's care. At the time of transportation, a member of the medical staff should be prepared to travel with the athlete to provide historical information and communication with not only the EMS but with the physicians taking over their care.

To ensure success, it would benefit all staff members, local emergency services, and hospitals to meet formally at designated intervals in the preseason period to review injury action plans and protocols. Throughout the season, all sporting event staff would also benefit from holding thorough pregame meetings to review the steps necessary to manage these situations, maximizing efficiency in the event of a serious injury. Preparation is key to successful management of an SCI, and although the treatment is complex, pregame preparation can help promote a safe and effective response.

INITIAL ON-FIELD MANAGEMENT

The on-field management of a potential spine injury is critical and begins from the sideline. Seeing the injury first-hand allows the team physician or staff to formulate a differential diagnosis based on the observed mechanism.[3] Extreme care must be taken in the first moments after the injury, as a patient may appear asymptomatic or be positioned in a way that is difficult to examine. It has been reported that up to 25% of SCIs are worsened under the care of medical professionals; although this may be an overestimation, it certainly emphasizes the importance of appropriate and safe management.[37] Therefore, avoidance of excessive movement is prudent, as it minimizes secondary injury to a potentially unstable spinal column.[38] Although it is rare that SCI will present with hemodynamic instability or cardiopulmonary arrest, Banerjee and colleagues[1,29,35] reported 3 presentations experienced by these athletes: (1) impending cardiopulmonary arrest, (2) altered mental status (AMS) with no imminent systemic threat, and (3) normal cardiopulmonary status and normal mentation.

As with any trauma, it is essential to evaluate the patient systemically through the use of basic life support (BLS)/advanced trauma life support (ATLS) algorithms following the "ABCDE sequence." A primary survey should always be conducted to assess for and rule out life-threatening injuries; first A, for airway management and cervical spine protection; B, breathing; C, circulation; D, disability (evaluating for any obvious neurologic deficits); E, exposure. Any indication of life-threatening or spinal injury should prompt immediate activation of EMS.

Cardiopulmonary compromise on the field can result from numerous etiologies. Although paralysis of the diaphragm may heighten suspicion of SCI; facial fractures, trauma to the trachea or larynx, foreign bodies, pneumothorax, and asthma exacerbations should be considered and managed appropriately if identified.[35] Regardless of the cause, the primary goal is to create a patent airway, ventilate the athlete, and begin cardiopulmonary resuscitation (CPR) if necessary.

In the event of a compromised airway, head tilt maneuvers should be avoided, as they can further propagate SCI. Instead, a jaw thrust maneuver should be used; this technique safely moves the tongue from the back of the throat, avoiding motion to the cervical spine, and permits access to the airway.[39] Ventilation is next provided via a bag-mask ventilation technique, if at this point the patient remains hypoxic, endotracheal intubation may be performed by a trained medical professional, again, remaining cognizant of spinal stability.[40] In the most severe cases, physicians should be capable of performing surgical airways if all other options fail.[3]

After securing an airway and confirming appropriate ventilation, the patient's circulatory status should be assessed. Diminished pulses and bradycardia or thready pulses and tachycardia may signify neurogenic or hypovolemic shock, respectively, with this, athletes require aggressive fluid resuscitation and strict maintenance of their mean arterial pressure at 85 mm Hg or greater to maintain spinal cord perfusion.[41] At this point, trained medical staff should be prepared to begin CPR and at any point in resuscitative efforts have an AED available in the event of hemodynamic collapse from irregular cardiac rhythms.

Protective padding may prevent efficient CPR or use of AEDs, whereas helmets should remain on the athlete with the chin strap in place if possible, chest pads can be safely removed by cutting straps or laces in the center of the padding near the chest or at the axilla to facilitate chest compressions. If this step is required during emergency stabilization, the medical provider in charge of the spine stabilization must remain cognizant of the aggressive resuscitative maneuver to avoid any changes in neck alignment. Additional challenges may present when an athlete is in a prone position, he or she should first be safely log rolled to the supine position followed by removal of any interfering protective equipment (management of protective equipment and movement of injured athletes is detailed in a later section) again with trained medical staff maintaining a neutral alignment to the cervical spine during the roll and through resuscitative efforts.

Once a patient's cardiopulmonary status is confirmed to be stable, a thorough assessment of the patient's level of consciousness should be performed. Physicians again must rely on observation, noting if a patient has any sporadic movements, postures, or even lack of movement, as this may clue one into central nervous system or spinal pathology. Signs of confusion and disorientation usually signify a sustained closed head injury and any signs of AMS should be considered in relation to an SCI until proven otherwise. The Glasgow coma scale (GCS) is a reliable and objective tool that may be used to evaluate an athlete's level of consciousness. The GCS assigns a score based on verbal cues, eye movement, and motor competency from 0 to 15, where a score of 11 or greater is reported to have a good to excellent prognosis and a score of 7 or less is associated with a poor prognosis.[42] Significant alteration in consciousness should warrant emergent medical evaluation regardless of the cause.

Finally, and most commonly, patients will present with normal mentation and no cardiopulmonary compromise. This does not exclude a catastrophic SCI, so the lead medical provider should maintain hypervigilant until a full evaluation has been performed. As these patients are able to communicate, they should remain motionless as an in-depth history is obtained by the physician. Any indication of neck pain (particularly midline), tenderness, limitations to motion, or bilateral neurologic compromise should warrant immediate immobilization and escalation of care.

STABILIZING THE INJURED SPINE FOR TRANSFER

In the event of a spine injury, it is recommended that a patient's neck be immobilized in neutral alignment before any movement.[43,44] If the injury has left the athlete's neck in an alternate position, it is acceptable to slowly correct the alignment of head and neck position to neutral, reassessing frequently, and stopping immediately with any change in pain or neurologic symptoms.[44] To stabilize the athlete's neck, the physician should be at the head of the athlete where he or she can cradle the occiput using their palms and fingertips to steady the mastoid processes bilaterally to bring the head and neck to the appropriate alignment.[45] The physician can then maintain this position as long as clinically necessary or until transition into a more rigid cervical collar. However, although a rigid cervical collar is effective to most injuries, complete ligamentous disruption requires the addition of continued manual stabilization due to the inherent instability of such injuries.[46]

Once a patient is safely immobilized in an appropriate cervical collar, the next step is to transfer the athlete to a backboard, to not only aid in further immobilization, but to prepare for transfer to the hospital setting. The task of moving an unstable spine should be handled delicately, as transfer to a backboard requires a perfect orchestration from the team leader and staff to move the head, neck, and body as a unit. Two maneuvers have been described to achieve this transfer: the lift and slide and the log roll techniques.

The lift and slide technique has been regarded as the preferred technique by the National Athletic Trainers Association (NATA) and confirmed on cadaveric studies, as it imparts less head and cervical spine motion compared with the log roll technique **(Fig. 1)**.[47,48] This procedure requires the injured athlete to be lifted off the ground approximately 6 inches in a neutral position permitting placement of the backboard. To accomplish this, a team of up to 8 people are required. In this technique, the team leader takes position at the patient's head so that he may dictate clear instruction to all assistants. The 6 additional people position themselves at the shoulders, pelvis, and at the lower extremities, 1 on each side of the athlete's body. The last individual is responsible for sliding the backboard beneath the patient before the athlete being safely lowered down and secured.

The log roll technique is performed similarly through direction of the team leader who again remains at, and is in charge of, the head and neck while providing instructions to those assisting. For this technique, the assistants are on the side the athlete is

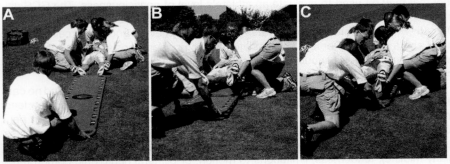

Fig. 1. The lift and slide technique. (*A*) The team leader remains at the head to stabilize the cervical spine and to verbalize all instructions to the assistants. Up to 7 additional assistants may be present and are positioned at the patient's shoulders, pelvis, and lower extremities bilaterally. (*B*) The patient is elevated in unison approximately 6 inches above the ground. (*C*) A final assistant slides the backboard beneath the elevated patient who is then slowly lowered onto it. (*From* Swartz EE et al. National Athletic Trainers' Association Position Statement: Acute Management of the Cervical Spine – Injured Athlete. J Athl Train. 2009; 44(3): 306-331, with permission.)

being rolled toward, in unison, the athlete is rolled up onto their side maintaining a neutral alignment from head to toe. The arms of the assistants should overlap across the athlete's body as they reach across, this allows for more stable points of fixation throughout the turn.[3] After the turn is completed and the board is placed under the athlete, the athlete is rolled back and secured to the board.

In the prone athlete, the log roll technique is required to turn the athlete into the supine position and also to permit the necessary primary survey. If possible, the log roll should be performed 1 time, meaning the patient is turned 180° and simultaneously placed onto a backboard directly (**Fig. 2**). However, this is not always attainable, if the athlete requires an emergent airway or CPR, expedient turning should be performed and the athlete can be transferred onto the backboard at a later time.[3] The technique is similar to the standard log roll described previously, a team leader at the head and a team of assistants uniformly turn the patient while minimizing motion to the head or neck with respect to the rest of the body. Overall, a team's medical staff should be familiar and well-practiced in both techniques, as limitations in personnel or situations may require the need to perform either technique.

MANAGING PROTECTIVE EQUIPMENT

Appropriate management of protective equipment on an athlete is of great importance in the event of a suspected SCI. Although helmets, face masks, and shoulder pads are

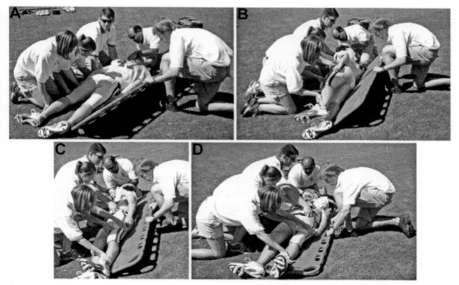

Fig. 2. The prone log roll technique. (*A*) The team leader remains at the head to stabilize the cervical spine leading the team through the maneuver. Additional assistants 2 to 4 position themselves on the side the athlete's head is facing. Assistant 5 is positioned on the opposite side to place the backboard. (*B*) Assistants 2 to 4 place their hands beneath the patient and roll on the command of the team leader toward assistant 5. (*C*) Assistant 5 places the backboard beneath the patient at a 45° angle as assistants 2 to 4 carefully turn the patient to the backboard. (*D*) The patient and backboard are lowed in unison to the ground. (*From* Swartz EE et al. National Athletic Trainers' Association Position Statement: Acute Management of the Cervical Spine – Injured Athlete. J Athl Train. 2009; 44(3): 306-331, with permission.)

designed to maintain a neutral cervical alignment and provide protection to the spine, medical providers must know how to not only stabilize an athlete in their equipment but also how to remove it. Helmets and facemasks can often interfere with a physican's primary survey, creating difficulty in the assessment of one's airway, breathing, and circulation. A decision to remove protective equipment should be based on numerous factors including the athlete's medical status at the time of injury, type of equipment being worn, and available trained medical staff.[49] All medical staff should have an in-depth understanding of the athletic equipment worn by all athletes, tools to disassemble or remove each piece of equipment, and appropriate training to do so. Pregame preparation and practice is key to minimize adverse events in dire situations.

In 2009, Swartz and colleagues[47] published the NATA Policy Statement with the goal of providing on-field medical providers with evidence-based recommendations in the event of injury. First, any suspicion of an SCI should be handled as if there is protective equipment or not with immobilization and stabilization followed by immediate BLS/ATLS protocols by a trained medical provider. When a facemask is present it can interfere with airway management and should be promptly removed with a tool and technique that minimizes or avoids excess motion to the neck.[47] During this process, at least 2 providers should be present, one to maintain head and neck control while the other removes the facemask. It is recommended that a cordless power screwdriver be used to remove the facemask from the helmet, as it can be quickly done and provides the least neck movement (**Fig. 3**).[50,51] In the event the facemask cannot be removed whether from damage during the injury or corrosion of the screws from equipment age/mismanagement, a backup tool to cut the facemask should always be available.[52,53] This also emphasizes the importance of frequent servicing of all athletic equipment to ensure safety to athletes and avoid complications in the emergent situations. If all methods of facemask removal fail and the situation is ominous, the facemask and helmet can be removed together by a team of trained providers. As always, the ultimate goal is to maintain neutral spine alignment throughout each step.[47]

Maintenance of helmets and shoulder pads have been widely studied and supported in the literature. By design, this equipment is meant to maintain spinal alignment and premature removal may exacerbate instability in the event of an SCI. Cadaveric studies by Palumbo and colleagues[54] and LaPrade and colleagues[55] examined cervical alignment after helmet removal and noted that there was increased risk of excessive neck extension, or hyperlordosis, which may exacerbate injury. It is preferred that the helmet and chin strap should remain in place unless it precludes management of the airway and proper immobilization. If necessary, removal of helmet and shoulder pads should be done simultaneously. Swenson and colleagues[56] demonstrated that removing them separately can elicit excessive motion and negatively impact spinal alignment.[6] For instance, maintaining the helmet and removing shoulder padding can accentuate flexion of the neck, where on the contrary removing the helmet and leaving the padding can lead to hyperextension.[3]

There are numerous circumstances that require prompt removal of protective gear on the field. First, if the protective gear is compromising the ability to perform a primary survey, particularly the assessment of an airway or ability to perform CPR or place an AED. Second, while a patient's helmet is usually used as a tool to stabilize, if the helmet is not properly fitted, using it to maintain head and neck alignment places the athlete in danger for exacerbation of injury. Finally, if the equipment is found to prevent a neutral or safe alignment of the spine, it should be removed expeditiously.[57,58]

The importance of safe equipment removal cannot be overemphasized. It is recommended by the NATA and the Inter-Association Task Force for Appropriate Care of the Spine-Injured Athlete that a 4-person technique should be implemented when

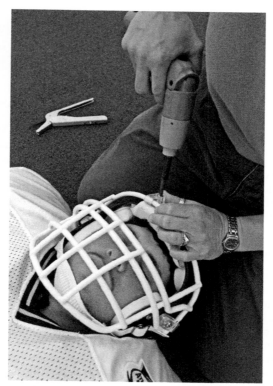

Fig. 3. Face-mask removal. The preferred technique is via a cordless power screwdriver while the head and neck alignment are maintained. This allows easy access to the airway while minimizing head and neck motion. (*From* Swartz EE et al. National Athletic Trainers' Association Position Statement: Acute Management of the Cervical Spine – Injured Athlete. J Athl Train. 2009; 44(3): 306-331, with permission.)

removing an athlete's helmet and shoulder pads. Peris and colleagues[59] went on to study this technique under dynamic fluoroscopy and showed that the 4-person technique effectively limited motion to the cervical spine. The 4-person technique is as follows: a team leader is at the head and responsible for removing the helmet and shoulder pads as the other 3 assistants lift the patient's body in unison. Another person is positioned at the neck, placing 1 hand anterior under the chin and 1 posterior behind the neck at the base of the occiput to stabilize it (**Fig. 4**). The other 2 assistants each place 1 hand under the scapula and the other to grab the ipsilateral arm. After the equipment has been removed, the patient should be placed in a rigid cervical collar before transfer to a backboard. Ultimately, this step would be preferred to occur after transport to the hospital with further help from medical personnel if the situation permits.

PEDIATRIC CONSIDERATIONS

The pediatric patient with a suspected SCI requires a similar management to that of an adult, first to rule out life-threatening injury and then immobilization of the neck in a neutral position. However, certain considerations must be made, during growth, the

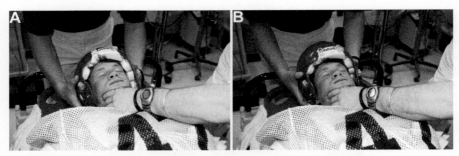

Fig. 4. Stabilization of the head and neck for helmet removal. (*A*) The team leader is positioned at the head with his or her hands on either side of the helmet. A second assistant places one hand anteriorly under the patient's chin and the other at the base of the occiput to stabilize the head and neck. (*B*) As the helmet is prepared for removal, 2 additional assistants (not pictured here) are recommended to lift the patient from the shoulder and ipsilateral extremity bilaterally so the equipment can be safely removed. (*From* Swartz EE et al. National Athletic Trainers' Association Position Statement: Acute Management of the Cervical Spine – Injured Athlete. J Athl Train. 2009; 44(3): 306-331, with permission.)

spine undergoes numerous changes between both bony and soft tissue structures predisposing it to unique injury patterns at different stages in development. As a person grows, delays in bone mineralization leave the spine susceptible to fracture secondary to its increased flexibility.[60] Also, during peak growth, soft tissues lag behind the accelerated growth of the bony anatomy and thereby create increased tension to the spine, which may predispose an athlete to injury.[31] Similar to adults, knowledge of injury patterns and mechanisms gives the medical staff the best information to appropriately manage these athletes.

On the field, pediatric injuries require additional training in airway management and movements during stabilization. Relative to adults, pediatric athletes will have a larger head to body ratio, which makes spinal immobilization and patient transportation unique. Due to the head being disproportionately larger to the body, placing the athlete on a flat board will result in exaggerated flexion of the neck, which can further exacerbate an SCI.[61] Therefore, it is required that the body be elevated in relation to the head, so the head and neck can rest in neural alignment. Pediatric spine boards are specifically designed to accommodate this, they have a depressed area for the head and padding to elevate the rest of the body from the shoulders distal. The recommended age for these backboards is 8 years or younger.[62]

PHARMACOLOGIC TREATMENT

In the initial moments after injury when the patient is medically stable and immobilized, there may be other treatment modalities that can benefit the athlete. At the primary traumatic event, the spinal cord undergoes significant compressive or contusing injury, and while this is unavoidable, research has focused on alleviating the "secondary injury" that may follow.[63] Secondary injury is defined as delayed injury to the spinal cord that elicits inflammation, ischemia, electrolyte imbalance, and lipid peroxidation, which ultimately contributes to spinal cord tissue death.[64] Although it is well known in the literature that time to surgical decompression can help mitigate additional neurologic deficits, pharmacologic therapy has been a topic of research in the immediate postinjury phase.

Corticosteroids have become a contentious topic as an adjunctive treatment in SCI. Specifically, methylprednisolone (MP), which initially gained favor after a series of 3 studies called the National Acute Spinal Cord Injury Studies I, II, and III (NASCIS). These were the first large clinical trials that reportedly demonstrated positive neurologic outcomes after high-dose MP treatment given within 8 hours of injury.[65–67] However, these studies quickly came under strong contention. The trials initially did not provide any data showing significant improvement in motor or sensory function but only after a post hoc analysis did small improvements in sensation result. In addition, high-dose MP is not without high risk of complications (septicemia, pneumonia, gastrointestinal bleeding, and cardiovascular disease), in the NASCIS trials, these studies were ultimately underpowered and unable to report these complications, which have been frequently cited in multiple other studies.[35,68]

In 2013, The American Association of Neurologic Surgeons and the Congress of Neurologic Surgeons Guidelines for the Management of SCI released level 1 evidence that MP is not recommended.[68] To follow, in 2019, a systematic review was performed by Liu and colleagues,[69] who evaluated 1863 patients over 16 studies who underwent MP use for acute SCI and concluded that MP was not associated with any significant improvement in outcome. In addition, they found patients did not have any increase in motor score, sensory recovery, or American Spinal Cord Injury Association (ASIA) grade with the added expense of significant adverse effects. Ultimately, they followed suit and continued the recommendation against the use of high-dose MP for the acute management of SCI.[69] This study was further confirmed by Sultan and colleagues[70] in 2020, who reviewed 12 studies and also noted significant complication from high-dose MP use with no short-term or long-term improvement in motor or sensory function. Although MP has demonstrated promise over years of study, at this time it is not recommended for on-field use of suspected SCI.

HYPOTHERMIA

The use of therapeutic hypothermia in the management of SCI has been investigated since the 1950s, but never gained traction due to its inconsistency in proper protocol and complications.[71] Although the exact mechanism is complex and not fully understood, animal studies have demonstrated histologic, biochemical, and pathophysiologic benefits toward secondary injury after the initial insult to the spine.[72] These potential benefits include reduced excitatory neurotransmitters in the cerebral spinal fluid, decreased vasogenic edema, decreased neutrophil count, and a lack of reduction in blood flow at the injured site.[73–75] Although these findings incite promise, many questions still remain: the target cooling temperature, duration of hypothermia, and rewarming protocols. Overall, until further clinical trials demonstrate data supporting defined and beneficial protocols in human subjects, hypothermia should not be recommended as an on-field intervention for suspected SCI.

DEFINITIVE MANAGEMENT

After an SCI, the time to surgical decompression is essential. Therefore on-field medical staff should have predetermined medical facilities to expedite and optimize the athlete's care. In 2012, the Surgical Timing In Acute Spinal Cord Injury Study (STASCIS), an international multi-centered prospective cohort study, compared early decompression within 24 hours vs late decompression after 24 hours of injury. This study concluded that surgical decompression within 24 hours was associated with an improvement of 2 ASIA grades in 19.8% of patients in comparison with only 8.8% of patients showing improvement when decompressed after 24 hours.[76] Overall, these are devastating injuries, and this study further emphasizes the need to have an appropriate on-field plan as early surgical decompression can optimize an athlete's outcome.

SUMMARY

SCI is an uncommon but devastating issue faced by athletes on the field. Although the acute management of these injuries is vitally important, it all begins with prevention and preparation. Before stepping out onto the field, the essential medical staff should be present as well as the appropriate equipment to manage a wide variety of injuries. Meetings should be held among all staff members before each event to review the predetermined algorithms necessary to treat suspected SCI. In these circumstances, communication among team members is key: a team leader should be predefined and each subsequent team member should be aware of their assigned role to maximize execution and minimize time to definitive management. At the time of injury, the team leader is responsible for the athlete's initial evaluation in accordance with BLS/ATLS protocols and spinal precaution; once the athlete is deemed stable, further evaluation and management can be performed. Although many other therapies such as steroid use and hypothermia have been investigated, clinical research at this time does not support their use in SCI on the field and should be avoided. Ultimately, any athlete with a suspected SCI requires prompt on-field spine immobilization, proper equipment management, and expedient transport to an SCI center to mitigate the risk of further injury.[77]

REFERENCES

1. Banerjee R, Palumbo MA, Fadale PD. Catastrophic cervical spine injuries in the collision sport athlete, part 2: principles of emergency care. Am J Sports Med 2004;32(7):1760–4.
2. National spinal cord injury statistical center, Facts and Figures at a Glance. Birmingham, AL: University of Alabama at Birmingham; 2020. Available at: https://www.nscisc.uab.edu/Public/Facts%20and%20Figures%202020.pdf. Accessed August 1, 2020.
3. Sahota S, Kelly B. On-field assessment and management of spine injuries. Spinal Conditions in the Athlete 2020;3–15. https://doi.org/10.1007/978-3-030-26207-5_1.
4. Nobunaga AI, Go BK, Karunas RB. Recent demographic and injury trends in people served by the model spinal cord injury care systems. Arch Phys Med Rehabil 1999;80(11):1372–82.
5. Torg JS. Epidemiology, pathomechanics, and prevention of athletic injuries to the cervical spine. Med Sci Sports Exerc 1985;17(3):295–303.
6. Sanchez AR 2nd, Sugalski MT, LaPrade RF. Field-side and prehospital management of the spine-injured athlete. Curr Sports Med Rep 2005;4(1):50–5.
7. Khan N, Husain S, Haak M. Thoracolumbar injuries in the athlete. Sports Med Arthrosc 2008;16(1):16–25.
8. Tator CH, Provvidenza C, Cassidy JD. Spinal injuries in Canadian ice hockey: an update to 2005. Clin J Sport Med 2009;19(6):451–6.
9. Cantu RC, Mueller FO. Catastrophic spine injuries in American Football, 1977–2001. Neurosurgery 2003;53(2):358–63.
10. Schroeder GD, Vaccaro AR. Cervical spine injuries in the athlete. Instr Course Lect 2017;66:391–402.

11. Torg JS, Quedenfeld TC, Burstein A, et al. National football head and neck injury registry: report on cervical quadriplegia, 1971 to 1975. Am J Sports Med 1979; 7(2):127–32.

12. Torg JS, Vegso JJ, O'Neill MJ, et al. The epidemiologic, pathologic, biomechanical, and cinematographic analysis of football-induced cervical spine trauma. Am J Sports Med 1990;18(1):50–7.

13. Matsuura P, Waters RL, Adkins RH, et al. Comparison of computerized tomography parameters of the cervical spine in normal control subjects and spinal cord-injured patients. J Bone Joint Surg 1989;71(2):183–8.

14. Eismont FJ, Clifford S, Goldberg M, et al. Cervical sagittal spinal canal size in spine injury. Spine 1984;9(7):663–6.

15. Torg JS, Naranja RJ Jr, Pavlov H, et al. The relationship of developmental narrowing of the cervical spinal canal to reversible and irreversible injury of the cervical spinal cord in football players. J Bone Joint Surg Am 1996;78(9):1308–14.

16. Aebli N, Rüegg TB, Wicki AG, et al. Predicting the risk and severity of acute spinal cord injury after a minor trauma to the cervical spine. Spine J 2013;13(6): 597–604.

17. Castro FP Jr. Stingers, cervical cord neurapraxia, and stenosis. Clin Sports Med 2003;22(3):483–92.

18. Meyer SA, Schulte KR, Callaghan JJ, et al. Cervical spinal stenosis and stingers in collegiate football players. Am J Sports Med 1994;22(2):158–66.

19. Tosti R, Rossy W, Sanchez A, et al. Burners, stingers, and other brachial plexus injuries in the contact athlete. Oper Tech Sports Med 2016;24(4):273–7.

20. Kawasaki T, Ota C, Yoneda T, et al. Incidence of stingers in young rugby players. Am J Sports Med 2015;43(11):2809–15.

21. Kelly JD 4th, Aliquo D, Sitler MR, et al. Association of burners with cervical canal and foraminal stenosis. Am J Sports Med 2000;28(2):214–7.

22. Markey KL, Di Benedetto M, Curl WW. Upper trunk brachial plexopathy. The stinger syndrome. Am J Sports Med 1993;21(5):650–5.

23. Weinberg J, Rokito S, Silber JS. Etiology, treatment, and prevention of athletic "stingers. Clin Sports Med 2003;22(3):493–500, viii.

24. Ahearn BM, Starr HM, Seiler JG. Traumatic brachial plexopathy in athletes: current concepts for diagnosis and management of stingers. J Am Acad Orthop Surg 2019;27(18):677–84.

25. Triantafillou KM, Lauerman W, Kalantar SB. Degenerative disease of the cervical spine and its relationship to athletes. Clin Sports Med 2012;31(3):509–20.

26. Gray BL, Buchowski JM, Bumpass DB, et al. Disc herniations in the national football league. Spine 2013;38(22):1934–8.

27. Yamaguchi JT, Hsu WK. Intervertebral disc herniation in elite athletes. Int Orthop 2019;43(4):833–40.

28. Lawrence JP, Greene HS, Grauer JN. Back pain in athletes. J Am Acad Orthop Surg 2006;14(13):726–35.

29. Banerjee R, Palumbo MA, Fadale PD. Catastrophic cervical spine injuries in the collision sport athlete, part 1. Am J Sports Med 2004;32(4):1077–87.

30. Boden BP, Tacchetti RL, Cantu RC, et al. Catastrophic cervical spine injuries in high school and college football players. Am J Sports Med 2006;34(8):1223–32.

31. Hecht A. Spine injuries in athletes. Lippincott Williams & Wilkins; 2017.

32. MacLean JGB, Hutchison JD. Serious neck injuries in U19 rugby union players: an audit of admissions to spinal injury units in Great Britain and Ireland. Br J Sports Med 2012;46(8):591–4.

33. Allen BL Jr, Ferguson RL, Lehmann TR, et al. A mechanistic classification of closed, indirect fractures and dislocations of the lower cervical spine. Spine 1982;7(1):1–27.
34. Vaccaro AR, Klein GR, Thaller JB, et al. Distraction extension injuries of the cervical spine. J Spinal Disord 2001;14(3):193–200.
35. Assenmacher B, Schroeder GD, Patel AA. On-field management of spine and spinal cord injuries. Oper Tech Sports Med 2013;21(3):152–8.
36. Macias CA, Rosengart MR, Puyana J-C, et al. The effects of trauma center care, admission volume, and surgical volume on paralysis after traumatic spinal cord injury. Ann Surg 2009;249(1):10–7.
37. Podolsky SM, Hoffman JR, Pietrafesa CA. Neurologic complications following immobilization of cervical spine fracture in a patient with ankylosing spondylitis. Ann Emerg Med 1983;12(9):578–80.
38. Bailes JE, Petschauer M, Guskiewicz KM, et al. Management of cervical spine injuries in athletes. J Athl Train 2007;42(1):126–34.
39. Criswell JC, Parr MJA, Nolan JP. Emergency airway management in patients with cervical spine injuries. Anaesthesia 1994;49(10):900–3.
40. Shatney CH, Brunner RD, Nguyen TQ. The safety of orotracheal intubation in patients with unstable cervical spine fracture or high spinal cord injury. Am J Surg 1995;170(6):676–80.
41. Vale FL, Burns J, Jackson AB, et al. Combined medical and surgical treatment after acute spinal cord injury: results of a prospective pilot study to assess the merits of aggressive medical resuscitation and blood pressure management. J Neurosurg 1997;87(2):239–46.
42. McAlindon RJ. On field evaluation and management of head and neck injured athletes. Clin Sports Med 2002;21(1):1–14, v.
43. Crosby ET. Airway management in adults after cervical spine trauma. Anesthesiology 2006;104(6):1293–318.
44. Swartz EE, Del Rossi G. Cervical spine alignment during on-field management of potential catastrophic spine injuries. Sports Health 2009;1(3):247–52.
45. Ching RP, Watson NA, Carter JW, et al. The effect of post-injury spinal position on canal occlusion in a cervical spine burst fracture model. Spine 1997;22(15):1710–5.
46. Horodyski M, Weight M, Conrad B, et al. Motion generated in the unstable lumbar spine during hospital bed transfers. J Spinal Disord Tech 2009;22(1):45–8.
47. Swartz EE, Boden BP, Courson RW, et al. National athletic trainers' association position statement: acute management of the cervical spine–injured athlete. J Athletic Train 2009;44(3):306–31.
48. Horodyski M, Conrad BP, Del Rossi G, et al. Removing a patient from the spine board: is the lift and slide safer than the log roll? J Trauma Inj Infect Crit Care 2011;70(5):1282–5.
49. Courson R, Ellis J, Herring SA, et al. Best practices and current care concepts in prehospital care of the spine-injured athlete in American Tackle Football March 2-3, 2019; Atlanta, GA. J Athl Train 2020;55(6):545–62.
50. Jenkins HL, Valovich TC, Arnold BL, et al. Removal tools are faster and produce less force and torque on the helmet than cutting tools during face-mask retraction. J Athl Train 2002;37(3):246–51.
51. Copeland AJ, Decoster LC, Swartz EE, et al. Combined tool approach is 100% successful for emergency football face mask removal. Clin J Sport Med 2007;17(6):452–7.

52. Swartz EE, Decoster LC, Norkus SA, et al. The influence of various factors on high school football helmet face mask removal: a retrospective, cross-sectional analysis. J Athl Train 2007;42(1):11.

53. Swartz EE, Norkus SA, Armstrong CW, et al. Face-mask removal: movement and time associated with cutting of the loop straps. J Athl Train 2003;38(2):120–5.

54. Palumbo MA, Hulstyn MJ, Fadale PD, et al. The effect of protective football equipment on alignment of the injured cervical spine. Am J Sports Med 1996;24(4):446–53.

55. LaPrade RF, Schnetzler KA, Broxterman RJ, et al. Cervical spine alignment in the immobilized ice hockey player. Am J Sports Med 2000;28(6):800–3.

56. Swenson TM, Lauerman WC, Blanc RO, et al. Cervical spine alignment in the immobilized football player. Radiographic analysis before and after helmet removal. Am J Sports Med 1997;25(2):226–30.

57. Donaldson WF 3rd, Lauerman WC, Heil B, et al. Helmet and shoulder pad removal from a player with suspected cervical spine injury. A cadaveric model. Spine 1998;23(16):1729–32 [discussion: 1732–3].

58. Prinsen RK, Syrotuik DG, Reid DC. Position of the cervical vertebrae during helmet removal and cervical collar application in football and hockey. Clin J Sport Med 1995;5(3):155–61.

59. Peris MD, Donaldson WFWF 3rd, Towers J, et al. Helmet and shoulder pad removal in suspected cervical spine injury: human control model. Spine 2002;27(9):995–8 [discussion: 998–9].

60. Steendijk R. Effect of puberty on rates of bone growth and mineralisation. Arch Dis Child 1980;55(8):655–6.

61. Herzenberg JE, Hensinger RN, Dedrick DK, et al. Emergency transport and positioning of young children who have an injury of the cervical spine. The standard backboard may be hazardous. J Bone Joint Surg Am 1989;71(1):15–22.

62. Nypaver M, Treloar D. Neutral cervical spine positioning in children. Ann Emerg Med 1994;23(2):208–11.

63. Kakulas BA. The clinical neuropathology of spinal cord injury. A guide to the future. Paraplegia 1987;25(3):212–6.

64. Bramlett HM, Dietrich WD. Progressive damage after brain and spinal cord injury: pathomechanisms and treatment strategies. Prog Brain Res 2007;161:125–41.

65. Efficacy of methylprednisolone in acute spinal cord injury. Ann Emerg Med 1984;13(9):745–6.

66. Bracken MB. Administration of methylprednisolone for 24 or 48 hours or tirilazad mesylate for 48 hours in the treatment of acute spinal cord injury. Results of the Third National Acute Spinal Cord Injury Randomized Controlled Trial. National Acute Spinal Cord Injury Study. JAMA 1997;277(20):1597–604.

67. Bracken MB, Shepard MJ, Collins WF, et al. A randomized, controlled trial of methylprednisolone or naloxone in the treatment of acute spinal-cord injury. Surv Anesthesiology 1991;35(1):50. https://doi.org/10.1097/00132586-199102000-00048.

68. Hurlbert RJ, Hadley MN, Walters BC, et al. Pharmacological therapy for acute spinal cord injury. Neurosurgery 2015;76(Suppl 1):S71–83.

69. Liu Z, Yang Y, He L, et al. High-dose methylprednisolone for acute traumatic spinal cord injury: A meta-analysis. Neurology 2019;93(9):e841–50.

70. Sultan I, Lamba N, Liew A, et al. The safety and efficacy of steroid treatment for acute spinal cord injury: A Systematic Review and meta-analysis. Heliyon 2020;6(2):e03414.

71. Ahmad FU, Wang MY, Levi AD. Hypothermia for acute spinal cord injury–a review. World Neurosurg 2014;82(1–2):207–14.
72. Batchelor PE, Skeers P, Antonic A, et al. Systematic review and meta-analysis of therapeutic hypothermia in animal models of spinal cord injury. PLoS One 2013; 8(8):e71317.
73. Yamamoto K, Ishikawa T, Sakabe T, et al. The hydroxyl radical scavenger Nicaraven inhibits glutamate release after spinal injury in rats. Neuroreport 1998;9(7): 1655–9.
74. Yu WR, Westergren H, Farooque M, et al. Systemic hypothermia following compression injury of rat spinal cord: reduction of plasma protein extravasation demonstrated by immunohistochemistry. Acta Neuropathol 1999;98(1):15–21.
75. Westergren H, Farooque M, Olsson Y, et al. Spinal cord blood flow changes following systemic hypothermia and spinal cord compression injury: an experimental study in the rat using Laser-Doppler flowmetry. Spinal Cord 2001;39(2): 74–84.
76. Fehlings MG, Vaccaro A, Wilson JR, et al. Early versus delayed decompression for traumatic cervical spinal cord injury: results of the Surgical Timing in Acute Spinal Cord Injury Study (STASCIS). PLoS One 2012;7(2):e32037. The Spine Journal. 2012;12(6):540.
77. Gale SD, Decoster LC, Swartz EE. The combined tool approach for face mask removal during on-field conditions. J Athl Train 2008;43(1):14–20.

Transient Quadriparesis and Cervical Neuropraxia in Elite Athletes

Wellington K. Hsu, MD[a,b,*]

KEYWORDS

- Transient quadriparesis • Cervical cord neurapraxia • Cervical cord neuropraxia
- Elite athlete • Professional athlete • Cervical stenosis

KEY POINTS

- Cervical spine injuries in the elite athlete present a unique conundrum for treatment, which depends on multiple factors including symptoms and type of sport played.
- Cervical stenosis is compatible with return-to-play even for collision sports as long as there is a minimum threshold of canal space and there are no significant clinical symptoms.
- Treatment and management of these conditions should be individualized based on athlete's career trajectory, symptoms, and potential future risks.

INTRODUCTION

Approximately 12,500 new cases of spinal cord injury (SCI) occur in the United States alone per year[1] with athletic participation accounting for 9%.[2] Although American football has lower rates of SCI than other sports, it remains the leading cause due to its relatively larger nationwide participation rates.[3] Hutton and colleagues recently estimated the rate of SCI in professional male Rugby Union players at approximately 4.1 per 100,000 player-hours with most of the injuries occurring during the collapse of the scrum, followed by making a tackle.[4] A cross-sectional study by Torg and colleagues demonstrated that out of 355 spinal injuries suffered at any level by Canadian hockey players, 20.8% experienced cervical spine injuries without associated SCI, whereas 12.9% had associated SCI.[5]

[a] Department of Orthopaedic Surgery, Northwestern University Feinberg School of Medicine, 676 North St. Clair Street, #1350, Chicago, IL 60611, USA; [b] Department of Neurological Surgery, Northwestern University Feinberg School of Medicine, 676 North St. Clair Street, #1350, Chicago, IL 60611, USA
* Department of Orthopaedic Surgery, Northwestern University Feinberg School of Medicine, 676 North St. Clair Street, #1350, Chicago, IL 60611.
E-mail address: whsu@nmff.org

Clin Sports Med 40 (2021) 463–470
https://doi.org/10.1016/j.csm.2021.03.003
0278-5919/21/© 2021 Elsevier Inc. All rights reserved.

Sports-related neurologic injuries can range in severity from stingers to catastrophic permanent neurologic injury. Stingers/burners are defined as a type of brachial plexopathy manifesting as transient sensory and/or motor deficits in the ipsilateral upper extremity resulting from compression- or traction-type trauma.[6] These injuries are differentiated from more severe spinal cord injuries by the unilateral nature of their symptoms, combined with painless active and passive neck range of motion (ROM). Even for these types of injuries, initial evaluation must rule out a more significant structural or SCI with formal work-up including cervical spine radiographs and MRI evaluation.

The incidence, management, and outcomes after major cervical spine injuries are of critical interest for athletes participating in collision sports. In particular, the management of athletes found to have cervical canal stenosis is a topic of considerable debate, with few definitive guidelines in place for such athletes' return to active play. The identification of cervical canal stenosis in athletes often occurs through imaging, following an injury with symptoms of neck pain, radiculopathy, or SCI. This condition can also be diagnosed during routine screening imaging in asymptomatic individuals. There is significant controversy in predicting the risk of future injury in athletes found to have cervical canal stenosis who are otherwise completely asymptomatic. Despite the prevalence of these conditions, there do not exist any standardized consensus guidelines for return-to-play (RTP). Many of the pertinent treatises for treatment in this population are based on expert opinion only. The diagnosis, management, and decision-making process surrounding cervical spinal injuries can be complex and must incorporate many different considerations—both short-term and long-term. The authors believe that large-scale retrospective cohort, case series, and even case report studies can be incorporated with expert opinion to set forth guidelines to practitioners and players who are afflicted by cervical spinal injuries.

TRANSIENT QUADRIPLEGIA

Transient quadriplegia is defined as a temporary loss of motor or sensory function in the arms and legs that can last from seconds to days following excessive compression, flexion, or extension injury of the cervical spine.[1,3,7–9] The presence of preexisting cervical stenosis greatly reduces functional reserve, which can increase the incidence of these symptoms with hyperextension or axial compression forces.[2] The severity of the episode also deserves consideration in the individualized RTP algorithm. The more severe and longer the duration of symptoms, the greater the ramifications and risk of neurologic sequelae with a repeat injury.

These types of injuries in athletes are primarily attributed to axial loading and hyperflexion mechanisms.[10] When the cervical spine is straightened with slight neck flexion (ie, checking, tackling, spearing), an applied axial load with sufficient energy can result in angular deformation and buckling, causing structural failures such as subluxations, fractures, and facet dislocations.[11] In adults, the subaxial spinal cord canal diameter from C4 to C7 is smaller than other regions, increasing the likelihood of SCI.[12] Furthermore, stenosis associated with "spear-tackling" has been shown to narrow the spinal canal as much as 30%.[13,14] Regardless of the mechanism, the potential for spinal cord irritation exists with each of these types of mechanisms and must be given particular attention. In many cases of transient quadriplegia, all 4 extremities are involved. The duration of symptoms typically lasts less than 15 minutes and can require up to 48 hours for the resolution of all symptoms.[9]

In a recent review, transient quadriplegia (n = 19 studies) occurred in 7.3 per 10,000 professional football players and was closely associated with the presence of congenital cervical stenosis, which puts the player at risk with extreme flexion and extension of the cervical spine.[4,5,8,10,15–18] Historically, Torg and colleagues suggested RTP recommendations for NFL athletes based on 0.8 vertebral canal-to-body ratio on plain radiographs and presence of symptoms. However, in a computed tomography (CT)-based evaluation of 80 NFL athletes, Herzog and colleagues demonstrated that nearly 50% of asymptomatic players had abnormal canal-to-body ratios, despite having average spinal canal measurements on advanced imaging.[11] These data challenge the specificity for the usage of this test in this patient population. More recent studies have identified the sagittal MRI as the most appropriate screening tool to diagnose cervical stenosis.[12,19] For example, the term "congenital cervical stenosis" has recently been specifically defined as a patient less than 50 years of age with midsagittal canal diameters of less than 10 mm at multiple subaxial cervical levels measured at the pedicle on MRI T2 imaging.[20] Furthermore, Aebli and colleagues recently reported that a sagittal canal diameter of less than 8 mm may increase the risk of SCI with minor trauma to the neck.[21] MRI evaluation can also lead to the qualitative diagnosis of stenosis, or "functional cervical spinal stenosis," that grades severity by the loss of protective cerebrospinal fluid (CSF) around the spinal cord.[17]

Cervical Cord Neuropraxia

Cervical cord neuropraxia (CCN), which is defined as the temporary cessation of spinal cord function after impact to the cervical region, is often the cause that leads to a transient quadriplegic episode. In counseling athletes presenting with prior reported incidents, it becomes important to discuss the risks of recurrence and permanent neurologic injury. One case series followed 110 patients who had a witnessed episode of CCN from a sports-related injury for an average follow-up of 40 ± 51 months.[9] Most of these patients (86%) were found to have radiographic cervical cord stenosis (Torg-Pavlov <0.8) with an average ratio of 0.68. MRI demonstrated an average minimum disc-level canal diameter of 9.6 mm and spinal cord diameter of 8.1 mm. A total of 63 of 110 patients returned to play, and of those, 56% reported a recurrence of CCN. Predictors of recurrence included playing American football, a smaller Torg-Pavlov ratio, a smaller disc-level canal diameter, and less space available for cord, which implicates cervical stenosis as a risk factor. Age, level of sport, and symptoms/severity of CCN were not found to be predictive of recurrence.[9]

Notably, no athlete followed in this study went on to suffer a permanent neurologic injury after returning to contact sports. Similarly, in other studies, athletes who had a football-related injury causing permanent quadriplegia denied any previous history of CCN.[13,14] This suggests that an episode of CCN, although a risk factor of recurrent episodes, is not associated with permanent neurologic injury. Thus, athletes without spinal instability who have had an episode of CCN are not at increased risk of permanent neurologic injury by returning to sport. This information can be valuable when discussing the risks of returning to play in athletes who have developmental cervical stenosis and a prior episode of CCN. It can also be inferred from the data that the more stenotic the individual's anatomy is, the more likely they are to have a recurrent episode; moreover, prediction of future injury can be made with evaluation of a sagittal MRI.

CERVICAL FRACTURES

Cervical fractures can occur when the area between the vertebral body and decelerating head undergoes rapid compression, requiring as little as 150 ft-lb of force to fracture the cervical vertebrae.[22–24] Certain fracture patterns involving the spinous process or unilateral lamina do not typically cause significant instability and require only hard-collar immobilization for a period of 6 to 12 weeks as definitive treatment.[25] Stability on flexion-extension radiographs after healing and maintenance of cervical lordosis are required for RTP.[22,24] Unstable fractures are best treated with surgical fixation,[24,26,27] and in general, the literature supports RTP for players who are treated with a one-level subaxial anterior or posterior fusion if there is no pain, full ROM, normal muscle strength, complete fusion on imaging, and a normal neurologic examination.[12]

Despite some disagreements, there seems to be strong consensus regarding certain absolute contraindications, including any patient with a fracture with residual neurologic deficits, underlying congenital stenosis, cervical laminectomy, and any procedures that require occipital, C1-C2, C2-C3, or 3+ level fusions.[24,28,29] Consideration for NFL athlete RTP should involve imaging demonstrating solid fusion in the area of injury, lack of instability on flexion and extension radiographs, maintenance of normal cervical lordosis, full ROM with no associated pain, and preinjury muscle strength.[24,25,28] In addition, sagittal misalignment greater than 11° when compared with other levels for isolated burst fractures and fractures that disrupt the posterior bony or ligamentous tension band may preclude RTP.[25,28]

Currently, expert opinions advocate that athletes can be cleared for a return to contact sports following cervical spine trauma after fulfilling the following conditions of full functional, pain-free ROM of the cervical spine, baseline muscle strength, and absence of neurologic deficits. A 2-level cervical fusion is considered a relative contraindication to return to athletic activity, whereas a three- or more level fusion is considered an absolute contraindication. Athletes who suffer a subaxial cervical spine fracture may be allowed to return to contact play depending on the morphology of the injury, its resultant stability at the time of healing, and neurologic status.

Absolute contraindications for return to athletic play in athletes with subaxial cervical spine injury include an association with a residual neurologic deficit and/or congenital stenosis. Relative contraindications for return to athletic play include healed compression and stable burst fractures of the subaxial cervical spine. Athletes with cervical spine stenosis or in the setting of a moderate-to-large disc herniation with a history of transient neuropraxia or quadriparesis should be counseled to avoid returning to contact play unless the focal stenosis can be surgically remedied. Finally, other absolute disqualification criteria include a history of 2 episodes of cervical spinal cord neuropraxia even in the absence of spinal stenosis and the "spear tackler's spine."[2]

Cervical Stenosis

There is a significant amount of controversy as it pertains to the diagnosis of cervical stenosis, which is defined as narrowing of the spinal canal.[30] Based on the available literature to date, the authors believe that practitioners should rely on 4 categories of information for the management of these conditions as it pertains to RTP: clinical symptoms, physical examination, sport and position played, and imaging characteristics.[31] In the setting of a player without any residual symptoms and normal strength and neurologic examination, individualized recommendations should rely on the type of demands of the player's respective sport as well as what the advanced imaging (eg, MRI) studies demonstrate. The categorization of collision (ie, American football, rugby, hockey, etc.) versus contact sports (basketball, soccer, lacrosse, etc.) is important because of the relative risk of repetitive and traumatic hyperextension and axial compression forces to the cervical spine. Collision sports such as American football, rugby, hockey, etc. represent a significantly higher risk of reinjury in players with stenosis than contact and noncontact sports.

Among plain radiographic measurements, the Torg-Pavlov ratio has historically been most commonly used to diagnose cervical stenosis, which compares the width of the spinal canal with the vertebral body on a lateral radiograph. The width of the spinal canal is measured by the sagittal diameter of the canal from the middle of the posterior vertebral body to the nearest point on the spinolaminar line. This measure has also been found to correlate with both the vertebral body-to-canal ratio seen on CT imaging and the vertebral body-to-CSF column ratio seen on MRI.[32] The threshold value that should be used to predict SCI is still under debate. Although the initial studies suggested that a ratio of 0.8 or lower was a significant predictor, Aebli and colleagues concluded that a threshold of 0.7 or less had the highest positive likelihood ratio to predict the occurrence of cervical spinal injury after minor trauma in the general population.[21] However, a threshold of 0.7 had a high specificity of 99% but also a low sensitivity of 51%. Notably, the Torg-Pavlov ratio was not predictive of severity of injury according to the ASIA criteria for those who did suffer SCIs in this study.[21]

Other measures have been used such as axial MRI images. In particular, 3 measurements have been implicated: the transverse spinal canal and cord area, the transverse and sagittal cord diameter, and the sagittal canal diameter of the cervical spine.[33] Ruegg and colleagues demonstrated that all of these values were less in those who suffered an SCI with the exception of cord area. Both a cord-canal-area ratio greater than 0.8 and space available for the cord less than 1.2 mm were found to reliably identify patients at risk for cervical SCI after minor cervical spine trauma.[33]

Based on the most recent literature, the authors believe that the measurement of the cervical spinal canal diameter on sagittal T2 MRI provides the most specific information in the diagnosis of this condition. Although historically cervical spinal stenosis had been defined as a space available for the cord less than 14 mm on plain radiographs,[34] more recent and pertinent data suggest that this threshold may be too conservative when it comes to the risk of an SCI in the elite athlete population. Despite a small sample size, recent data suggest that 10-mm sagittal canal diameter measured on MRI is compatible with successful American football careers without increased risk of neurologic sequelae.[35] Furthermore, Aebli and colleagues demonstrated that sagittal canal diameter of less than 8 mm on MRI increases the risk of acute SCI after minor trauma to the cervical spine.[21] Although there are certainly other data that use other measures of spinal canal space,[36] most of the evidence-based literature points toward this range as a potential threshold for RTP criteria when treating these athletes. In a systematic review of clinical studies involving high-energy contact athletes, Dailey and colleagues strongly recommended that those without stenosis can return to play and weakly recommended those with stenosis not to return to play after one episode of transient cervical cord neurapraxia.[8]

RECOMMENDATIONS

The decision to return to play to both contact and collision sports with cervical stenosis is a complicated one for the athlete, family, and physician alike. Certain radiographic and MRI criteria may be helpful in identifying cervical stenosis. In particular, using plain radiographs, a Torg-Pavlov ratio less than 0.7 yields the highest positive predictive value for cervical SCI. Further MRI criteria such as the minimal disc-level canal diameter less than 8 mm, a cord-canal-area ratio greater than 0.8, or space available for the cord less than 1.2 mm can also be valuable for diagnosis. These 3 criteria may identify the "at-risk" athlete for more severe consequences and allow other athletes with measurements greater than these levels to return back to sport. For asymptomatic athletes without any previous neurologic deficits with space available for the cord greater than these thresholds, it is likely safe for them to return to both contact and collision sports.

For patients with cervical stenosis who have had an episode of cervical cord neuropraxia, counseling can be a critical asset. After a CCN without cervical stenosis or instability, the player may safely return to play once neurologically normal and demonstrate full painless range of motion. When CCN is associated with space available for the cord lower than published thresholds, there is some disagreement among practitioners in the management of these athletes. Although most would recommend not to return to collision sports after a second episode of a CCN with cervical stenosis, there have not been any cases documenting permanent neurologic or SCI after RTP. Especially for patients in high-risk sports, such as American football and rugby, counseling patients about the possibility of recurrence is very important.

Absolute contraindications of RTP[15] include persistent neurologic symptoms, cervical pain, loss of ROM, os odontoideum, basilar invagination, atlanto-occipital instability, Chiari malformation, functional spinal stenosis, cervical instability due to fracture or ligamentous disruption, symptoms lasting greater than 36 hours, or repeat episodes of transient quadriplegia.[3,15,25] RTP recommendations in American football athletes who demonstrate persistent cord hyperintensity (myelomalacia) despite surgical treatment is controversial.[37] Spinal cord signal changes in T1- or T2-weighted MRI sequences (hypo-/hyperintense areas with focal atrophy) can be an indicator of persistent swelling and parenchymal disruption of the spinal cord. Although the presence of residual edema in the spinal cord may represent smaller reserve to withstand future forces on the cervical spine, Maroon and colleagues recommends that cord hyperintensity after surgery may not preclude RTP in NFL athletes.[19,38] Tempel and colleagues also reported persistent T2 hyperintensity in 3 professional athletes, all of whom returned to play without reinjury.[19] Nonetheless, the presence of residual cord signal changes even in the absence of cervical stenosis or a herniated disc remains a relative contraindication for RTP.

SUMMARY

In summary, RTP indications for patients with a history of congenital cervical stenosis or transient quadriplegia are controversial. Imaging studies should be considered in context with the athlete's history, mechanism of injury, physical examination, and discussion of specific RTP risks with the athletes.[12,26,39] Most athletes with cervical stenosis and 2 episodes of CCN usually do not return to contact sports. Athletes with an episode of a CCN with a defined lesion such as a disc herniation can often have surgical treatment that allows successful RTP.

DISCLOSURE

The author has nothing to disclose.

REFERENCES

1. Naden CM. Brachial plexopathy. Curr Sports Med Rep 2017;16(3):121.
2. Mayer JE, Cho SK, Qureshi SA, et al. Cervical spine injury in athletes. Curr Orthop Pract 2012;23(3):181–7.
3. Rosenthal BD, Boody BS, Hsu WK. Return to play for athletes. Neurosurg Clin N Am 2017;28(1):163–71.

4. Dailey A, Harrop JS, France JC. High-energy contact sports and cervical spine neuropraxia injuries: what are the criteria for return to participation? Spine 2010;35(21 Suppl):S193.
5. Torg JS, Corcoran TA, Thibault LE, et al. Cervical cord neurapraxia: classification, pathomechanics, morbidity, and management guidelines. J Neurosurg 1997; 87(6):843.
6. Rihn J, Anderson D, Lamb K, et al. Cervical spine injuries in american football. Sports Med 2009;39(9):697–708.
7. Torg JS, Sennett B, Pavlov H, et al. Spear tackler's spine. An entity precluding participation in tackle football and collision activities that expose the cervical spine to axial energy inputs. Am J Sports Med 1993;21(5):640–9.
8. Cantu R. Current thinking: return to play and transient quadriplegia. Curr Sports Med Rep 2005;4(1):27–32.
9. Penning L. Some aspects of plain radiography of the cervical spine in chronic myelopathy. Neurology 1962;12:513.
10. Brigham CD, Adamson TE. Permanent partial cervical spinal cord injury in a professional football player who had only congenital stenosis. A case report. J Bone Joint Surg Am 2003;85(8):1553.
11. Wolf BS, Khilnani M, Malis L. The sagittal diameter of the bony cervical spinal canal and its significance in cervical spondylosis. J Mount Sinai Hosp 1956; 23(3):283.
12. Morganti C, Sweeney CA, Albanese SA, et al. Return to play after cervical spine injury. Spine 2001;26(10):1131.
13. Torg JS. Cervical spine injuries and the return to football. Sports Health 2009;1(5): 376–83.
14. Grant TT, Puffer J. Cervical stenosis: a developmental anomaly with quadriparesis during football. The Am J Sports Med 1976;4(5):219–21.
15. Herzog RJ, Wiens JJ, Dillingham MF, et al. Normal cervical spine morphometry and cervical spinal stenosis in asymptomatic professional football players. Plain film radiography, multiplanar computed tomography, and magnetic resonance imaging. Spine (Phila Pa 1976) 1991;16(6 Suppl):S178–86.
16. Tempel ZJ, Bost JW, Norwig JA, et al. Significance of T2 hyperintensity on magnetic resonance imaging after cervical cord injury and return to play in professional athletes. Neurosurgery 2015;77(1):23–30, discussion 30-21.
17. Brigham CD, Capo J. Cervical spinal cord contusion in professional athletes: a case series with implications for return to play. Spine 2013;38(4):315.
18. Jenkins TJ, Mai HT, Burgmeier RJ, et al. The triangle model of congenital cervical stenosis. Spine (Phila Pa 1976) 2016;41(5):E242–7.
19. Aebli N, Ruegg TB, Wicki AG, et al. Predicting the risk and severity of acute spinal cord injury after a minor trauma to the cervical spine. Spine J 2013;13(6): 597–604.
20. Boden BP, Tacchetti RL, Cantu RC, et al. Catastrophic cervical spine injuries in high school and college football players. Am J Sports Med 2006;34(8):1223–32.
21. Torg JS, Naranja RJ Jr, Pavlov H, et al. The relationship of developmental narrowing of the cervical spinal canal to reversible and irreversible injury of the cervical spinal cord in football players. J Bone Joint Surg Am 1996;78(9):1308–14.
22. Bailes JE, Petschauer M, Guskiewicz KM, et al. Management of cervical spine injuries in athletes. J Athletic Train 2007;42(1):126.
23. Torg JS, Vegso JJ, O'Neill MJ, et al. The epidemiologic, pathologic, biomechanical, and cinematographic analysis of football-induced cervical spine trauma. Am J Sports Med 1990;18(1):50–7.

24. Cantu RC, Li YM, Abdulhamid M, et al. Return to play after cervical spine injury in sports. Curr Sports Med Rep 2013;12(1):14.
25. Paulus S, Kennedy DJ. Return to play considerations for cervical spine injuries in athletes. Phys Med Rehabil Clin N Am 2014;25(4):723–33.
26. Maroon JC, Bailes JE. Athletes with cervical spine injury. Spine 1996;21(19):2294.
27. Rodts GE, Baum GR, Stewart FG, et al. Motion-preserving, 2-stage transoral and posterior treatment of an unstable Jefferson fracture in a professional football player. J Neurosurg Spine 2018;28(2):149–53.
28. Schroeder GD, Vaccaro AR. Cervical spine injuries in the Athlete. J Am Acad Orthop Surg 2016;24(9):e122.
29. Puvanesarajah V, Qureshi R, Cancienne JM, et al. Traumatic sports-related cervical Spine injuries. Clin Spine Surg 2017;30(2):50.
30. France JC, Karsy M, Harrop JS, et al. Return to play after cervical spine injuries: a consensus of opinion. Glob Spine J 2016;6(8):792–7.
31. Pahapill RR. Controversies in the managemetn of cervical spine conditions in Elite Athletes. J Orthopaedics 2019;42(4):e370–5.
32. Suk KS, Kim KT, Lee JH, et al. Reevaluation of the Pavlov ratio in patients with cervical myelopathy. Clin Orthop Surg 2009;1(1):6–10.
33. Ruegg TB, Wicki AG, Aebli N, et al. The diagnostic value of magnetic resonance imaging measurements for assessing cervical spinal canal stenosis. J Neurosurg Spine 2015;22(3):230–6.
34. Boden SD, Dodge LD, Bohlman HH, et al. Rheumatoid arthritis of the cervical spine. A long-term analysis with predictors of paralysis and recovery. J Bone Joint Surg Am 1993;75(9):1282–97.
35. Schroeder GD, Lynch TS, Gibbs DB, et al. The impact of a cervical spine diagnosis on the careers of National Football League athletes. Spine (Phila Pa 1976) 2014;39(12):947–52.
36. Bailes JE. Experience with cervical stenosis and temporary paralysis in athletes. J Neurosurg Spine 2005;2(1):11–6.
37. Milles JL, Gallizzi MA, Sherman SL, et al. Does a syrinx matter for return to play in contact sports? a case report and evidence-based review of return-to-play criteria after transient quadriplegia. Sports Health 2014;6(5):440–5.
38. Maroon JC, Bost JW, Petraglia AL, et al. Outcomes after anterior cervical discectomy and fusion in professional athletes. Neurosurgery 2013;73(1):103–12, discussion 112.
39. Maroon JC. Burning hands' in football spinal cord injuries. JAMA 1977;238(19):2049.

Lumbosacral Spondylolysis and Spondylolisthesis

Christopher C. Chung, BS, Adam L. Shimer, MD*

KEYWORDS

- Athlete • Spondylolysis • Spondylolisthesis • Pars interarticularis • Return to activity
- Pars stress reaction

KEY POINTS

- Pars injury is a common cause of back pain in the athletic population, particularly in adolescents and young adults.
- MRI is a potential alternative to computed tomography/single-photon emission computed tomography for initial diagnostic imaging of pars injury.
- Conservative management with rest and rehabilitation is the mainstay for treatment of pars defects.
- Surgical intervention may be considered after 6 to 12 months of failed conservative management or in cases of severe spondylolisthesis or progressive neurologic deficit.

PATHOPHYSIOLOGY AND INCIDENCE

Spondylolysis describes the fracture defect in the pars interarticularis of the lumbar vertebrae, which may be found as a unilateral or bilateral lesion. One or more vertebral levels may be involved, with the L5 vertebrae most commonly injured in spondylolysis. Bilateral pars defects may lead to progressive anterior translation of the involved vertebrae relative to the next caudal level, termed spondylolisthesis. Thus, the injury pattern of the pars exists on a spectrum, from stress reactions detected by advanced imaging methods to full anterior vertebral subluxation or spondyloptosis.

The pathophysiological development of pars injury may be multifactorial, as some studies suggest there is a genetic predisposition to spondylolysis.[1-3] However, the predominant contributing factor, particularly relevant to the athletic individual, is the force exerted on the lumbar pars by repetitive hyperextension, axial loading, and rotational motion with sporting activities. The repetitive stress pattern initiates a cycle of microfracture and healing in the pars, until cortical defects arise from a failure of bony remodeling. The notion that physical activity contributes to the development

Department of Orthopaedic Surgery, University of Virginia, PO Box 800159, Charlottesville, VA 22908, USA
* Corresponding author.
E-mail address: ALS5C@hscmail.mcc.virginia.edu

Clin Sports Med 40 (2021) 471–490
https://doi.org/10.1016/j.csm.2021.03.004
0278-5919/21/© 2021 Elsevier Inc. All rights reserved.

sportsmed.theclinics.com

of spondylolysis is supported by the 0% prevalence found in nonambulatory patients.[4] Further, young athletes have a higher prevalence of pars defect compared with nonathletes.[5]

The incidence of pars defects arising from such repetitive microtrauma in children is 4.4% by 6 years of age and increases to 6% by 18 years.[6] Although many cases are asymptomatic, spondylolysis and spondylolisthesis are commonly identified as the cause of lower back pain in the adolescent population.[7,8] Pars injury has classically been associated with gymnasts, but athletes in other sports including wrestling, rowing, diving, weight-lifting, and throwing sports have also demonstrated a high prevalence of pars injury.[9–11] In addition, multiple case series have reported on spondylolysis management for athletes competing in tennis, soccer, cricket, and volleyball, among other sports.[12–15] For the athletic adolescent patient presenting with lower back pain, injury to the pars should be given strong consideration when working up the differential diagnosis.

CLASSIFICATION

The Wiltse-Newman classification was described in 1976, grouping spondylolisthesis into different categories.[16] Type I, termed dysplastic spondylolisthesis, describes the abnormal congenital development of lumbosacral articulation, predisposing the L5 vertebral body to slip anteriorly relative to the sacrum over time. Type II, or isthmic, spondylolisthesis occurs as a result of a defect in the pars interarticularis and is subcategorized into 3 groups. Type IIA describes the isthmic fatigue fracture arising from repetitive loading and microtrauma to the pars interarticularis. Type IIB includes isthmic fractures that occur after elongation of the pars from the cyclic incidence of stress fractures and bony healing. Notably, this type of injury pattern can be difficult to distinguish from dysplastic spondylolisthesis. Type IIC describes pars fracture after an acute injury.[16] Type I and II spondylolisthesis are more relevant for consideration in the athletic population, particularly for children and adolescents.

Several other classifications describing spondylolisthesis have been created without widespread adoption. Marchetti and Bartolozzi developed a separate classification system, which divides spondylolisthesis broadly into 2 categories, developmental or acquired.[17] The Meyerding classification describes the percent slippage of the proximal vertebral body.[18] More recent classifications were created by combining components of Wiltse-Newman with Marchetti and Bartolozzi to guide nonoperative treatment and surgical management.[19–21]

CLINICAL EVALUATION

A thorough history and comprehensive physical examination should be conducted during the initial encounter with athletic patients. Patients with spondylolysis often present with insidious onset of lower back pain associated with motions required for sporting activity. The pain may occasionally radiate to the buttocks or lower extremities, although neurologic symptoms and deficits are rare findings with spondylolysis. Patients will report modifications in activity participation to accommodate the pain, and some may find their symptoms to interfere with other daily activities. Clarifying the timeline of symptomatic progression may assist with diagnosis in consideration of other organic causes for low back pain, including sacroiliac dysfunction or lumbar disk herniation. Other questions directed at dietary and nutritional intake may elucidate an increased risk for bony fracture.[22] The implementation of social needs screening may also identify barriers to maintaining nutritional needs in the growing adolescent, which should be addressed with all families regardless of perceived socioeconomic status.[23]

The physical examination begins with inspection for spinal deformity and other superficial abnormalities. Many reports have associated scoliosis and spina bifida occulta with an increased risk of lumbar spondylolysis.[24–28] Tenderness and spasms over the paraspinal regions may also contribute to apparent spinal curvature.[19] Lumbar range of motion may be limited particularly in lumbar flexion and extension, with pain often elicited with hyperextension. Single-leg hyperextension, or the stork test, can accentuate the pain.[7,29] Patients will frequently experience hamstring tightness, which may affect changes in gait.[19] Spondylolisthesis may also be suspected in patients with a vertically oriented sacrum and visible or palpable vertebral step-off. No clinical maneuvers have demonstrated high sensitivity or specificity for the diagnosis of pars injury,[30,31] but a high index of suspicion from the clinical history and examination should prompt further investigation with diagnostic imaging modalities.

DIAGNOSTIC IMAGING
Radiography

Prompt diagnostic imaging plays an important role in the prognosis and treatment of athletes, as pars injuries identified in the acute phase of development have shown better healing with conservative management.[32] Standard anteroposterior and lateral radiographic views are typically acquired as a part of initial screening to assess obvious bony pathology. The lateral view is also used to describe the severity of anterior slippage in spondylolisthesis, with less than 50% translation (Meyerding I or II) considered low-grade and Meyerding III–V as high-grade.[18] However, standard radiographs have demonstrated a low sensitivity in the diagnosis of pars defects. Oblique spinal views (**Fig. 1**) are often acquired to demonstrate the classic "Scotty dog sign,"[33] although recent studies have demonstrated poor diagnostic utility of oblique views.[34,35] The lucent defect described as the dog collar is seen most reliably only in late-stage spondylolysis, such that a negative radiograph cannot exclude early stage stress fractures.[35] Despite these limitations, radiographic imaging is frequently obtained because it remains a relatively affordable and accessible measure for initial screening.

Computed Tomography

Standard axial and sagittal computed tomography (CT) of the lumbar spine provides excellent resolution of the bony anatomy to characterize cortical defects, incomplete fractures, and sclerotic changes associated with pars injury.[36,37] Even modified protocols, with comparable radiation exposure to plain radiography, outperform standard radiographic imaging in the diagnosis of spondylolysis.[38] Plain CT images are superior in demonstrating disruptions to bony cortex, with early pars fractures typically identified as defects in the inferior margin and subsequent extension to the superior margin found as the fracture progresses (**Fig. 2**A, B).[39] CT imaging is also used to assess fracture healing.[40] However, the limitation with CT, particularly in comparison with single-photon emission CT (SPECT) and MRI, is the inability to identify early stress reactions[40,41] and to distinguish acute from chronic injury patterns.[42]

Single-Photon Emission Computed Tomography

The acquisition of single-photon emission computed tomography (SPECT) involves the intravenous injection of radioisotopes to identify regions with high rates of bony turnover. Metabolically active sites of stress fracture can be identified earlier in the

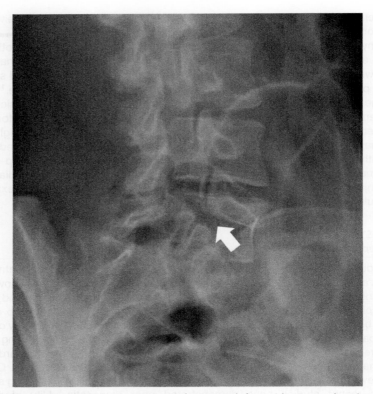

Fig. 1. Oblique radiograph demonstrating left L5 pars defect with "Scotty dog sign" (*white arrow*) in an adolescent gymnast.

progression of injury with SPECT compared with radiography or CT (**Fig. 2**C, D).[42–46] However, radiotracer uptake in posterior elements of the spine is nonspecific for pars injury and may reflect an active secondary ossification center, vertebral pedicle fracture, infection, or developing neoplasm.[45,47] In the athletic population, asymptomatic patients with spondylolysis have had positive radionuclide imaging,[48] and some symptomatic patients with positive SPECT have no demonstrated signs of pars injury on CT.[49] Although some have advocated for the hybrid acquisition of SPECT and CT to increase the combined diagnostic utility,[47,50,51] others find the false-positive and false-negative rate of SPECT too high to justify its use as a primary screening modality, particularly given the increased cost and radiation exposure to patients.[39,40,52,53]

MRI

MRI has recently emerged as a potential alternative to CT or SPECT for initial diagnostic imaging of suspected lumbosacral spondylolysis. A major benefit with the use of MRI is the avoidance of radiation exposure, which is particularly relevant for young, skeletally immature athletes. MRI provides insight into anatomic structures, with better soft tissue visualization, and is able to characterize activity changes at the pars interarticularis.[54,55] Although abnormalities on MRI are detected in asymptomatic patients,[56–58] MRI may be helpful in identifying other contributing factors to lower back pain besides spondylolysis.[55] In addition, although CT is considered the

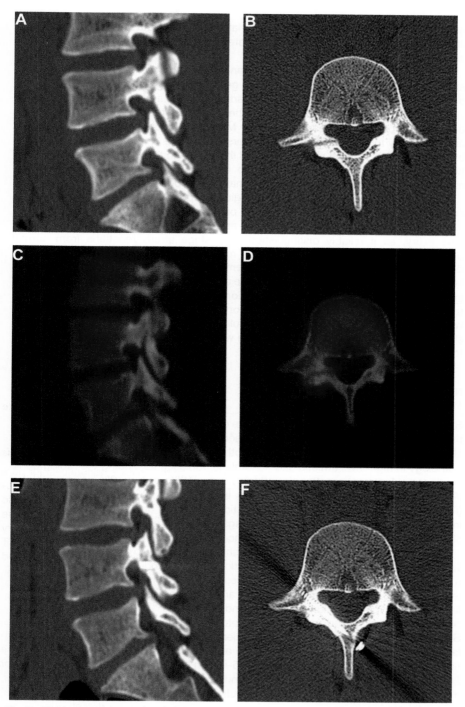

Fig. 2. CT (*A, B*) and SPECT (*C, D*) demonstrating a right L4 pars interarticularis defect in an elite-level football player. Postoperative CT imaging after percutaneous Buck screw fixation through the unilateral defect (*E, F*).

gold standard for evaluation of osseous anatomy, recent data also suggest that specific MRI sequences can detect incomplete and complete pars fractures with high accuracy.[59,60]

Hollenberg and colleagues[61] used T1- and T2-weighted sagittal and T2-weighted axial sequences for lumbosacral MRI to generate a 5-grade classification system describing stress reaction at the pars interarticularis. The addition of a short-tau inversion recovery sequence also improves the sensitivity for bone marrow edema to detect early pars stress reactions.[39,62,63] MRI has demonstrated a high sensitivity and specificity for distinguishing normal pars from grade 1 or higher injury, comparable to bone SPECT.[40,52] It should be noted that although there exists discrepancy between results using SPECT and MRI to detect stress reactions, the 2 imaging modalities identify distinctly separate biomarkers for bone stress.[39]

With multiple options for advanced imaging of spondylolytic defects, there is little consensus on the appropriate diagnostic pathway. In recent years, there has been increasing momentum for the use of MRI as the first-line imaging test in suspected pars injury, as it reliably distinguishes early stage stress reactions from normal pars.[39,40,52] Evaluation with CT and SPECT may be more warranted to guide treatment decisions in the case of refractory management or for athletes in high-level competition. Regardless of diagnostic modality, the ultimate goal of management for spondylolysis and spondylolisthesis is the alleviation of debilitating symptoms and the return to preinjury activity. Because osseous union on imaging has shown poor correlation with clinical outcomes,[64–66] the use of follow-up imaging to demonstrate healing should be avoided in patients progressing with rehabilitation protocols and reserved for those with refractory symptoms.

NONOPERATIVE MANAGEMENT
Stress Reactions

Stress injuries of the pars interarticularis are commonly found in athletes. A retrospective analysis of adolescent athletes with acute low back pain found a spondylolytic stress fracture in 47% of their cohort.[7] Another retrospective study compared lumbar pathology in high-level athletic and nonathletic adolescents, finding the radiographic incidence of stress reaction in athletes was 12% versus 2% in nonathletes ($P = .08$), with spondylolysis occurring in 32% and 2% in respective cohorts ($P = .0003$).[67] Because cortical stress reactions are better delineated by CT or SPECT imaging, having a high suspicion with negative radiographic findings in an athlete should prompt further work-up with advanced imaging.

Athletes with pars stress reactions have shown a capacity to heal and return to sport with early rest from activity and immobilization. Jackson and colleagues[29] reported on a case series of 7 athletes with pars stress reaction who returned to sport at an average of 7.3 months after initial resting and variable use of a form-fitting brace to limit lumbar hyperextension. Anderson and colleagues[68] followed 34 patients with pars stress reaction and found that symptomatic alleviation and improvements on SPECT studies were more robust in the patients initiated on early bracing. Sys and colleagues[66] initiated bracing for competitive athletes with spondylolytic defects identified by positive bone scan, leading to 5.5-month average return to competition for 25/28 of their cohort. Early recognition and therapy lead to better osseous healing and can prevent the progression of stress reaction to the development of spondylolysis.[13,48,69]

Despite a general consensus regarding restriction of activity to promote early bony healing and progressive return to play, specific protocols for management of pars stress reaction are likely derived from more prevalent literature on rehabilitation for spondylolysis and spondylolisthesis. The senior author's approach to athletic patients with pars stress reactions involves 6 to 12 weeks of rest from activity, without external bracing for immobilization. Physical therapy is initiated after the initial period of rest with an individualized timeline for return to activity based on symptomatic resolution and other patient-specific factors. The physical therapy program is focused on strengthening of deep core musculature while limiting hyperextension of the lumbosacral junction.

Spondylolysis

Conservative management is the mainstay of treatment of diagnosed spondylolysis in the athletic patient. A period of rest from activity is indicated typically until, at least, the patient experiences alleviation of pain, although some investigators suggest a minimum 3 months of restriction from sport.[12,70–73] Targeted physical therapy is generally recommended, with exercises directed at deep abdominal musculature and lumbar multifidi contributing to improvements in pain and functional outcome.[74] However, the timing for introduction of physical therapy is variable in the literature, with some advocating for early therapy[75–77] and others recommending that rehabilitation start after the initial period of activity restriction.[71,73] Selhorst and colleagues[77] conducted a retrospective analysis of adolescents who were referred to physical therapy before or after 10 weeks of rest from activity and found faster return to activity with earlier initiation of physical therapy. Recommendations on timing for rehabilitation are based on low-level evidence and generally derive from anecdotal physician practices.

The utility of bracing for spondylolysis remains a controversial topic. Several studies have reported on successful outcomes for return to activity with different braces, including thoracolumbosacral orthotics and lumbosacral orthotics.[48,65,66,76,78–81] However, a meta-analysis of studies using lumbar bracing identified no difference in clinical outcomes associated with usage,[64] and bracing did not prognosticate poor long-term outcomes.[82] Biomechanical studies have suggested that lumbar bracing is less effective at stabilizing the lower intervertebral segments that are most commonly involved in isthmic spondylolysis.[83,84] True immobilization at L5 and S1 is achieved only with the use of a leg extension, and its use is rarely reported in the literature. Confounding the proposed benefits of spinal stabilization and motion restriction may be a general adherence to activity restriction. For these reasons, the senior author's general approach is conservative therapy without bracing initially, with reconsideration for use in those patients whose symptoms are persistent after 6 to 12 weeks.

The concept of osseous union or healing of the spondylosis is an intuitively attractive one, but the rate of lysis healing is in actuality quite low. In a meta-analysis of 10 radiographic studies, Klein and colleagues[64] found that only 28% of spondylolytic lesions healed. Furthermore, multiple studies have shown no correlation with osseus union and clinical outcomes.[64–66] Therefore, the goal of treatment of spondylolysis is symptomatic alleviation, rather than osseous healing on imaging. For the clinically improving athlete, it is unnecessary to demonstrate radiographic healing, thereby avoiding radiation exposure and the associated costs of further imaging.[85]

Spondylolisthesis

Nonsurgical management of low-grade isthmic spondylolisthesis in athletes is frequently treated similarly as spondylolysis. Several studies on conservative management of spondylolysis also included patients with grade-I spondylolisthesis in their cohort analysis.[7,66,79,81] Pizzutillo and Hummer demonstrated pain relief in two-thirds of patients with grade 2 or lower slippage, whereas all 28 patients in a case series by Bell and colleagues were pain free after brace treatment.[78,80] Similar to the strategy for patients with spondylolysis, rest from activity and rehabilitation should be prioritized to alleviate pain and hamstring spasm with progressive return to sport based on individual response to therapy.

Several studies on the natural history of spondylolisthesis demonstrate a low rate of progression in adolescent populations (**Fig. 3**).[86–88] However, the rate of slippage may be slightly increased in the athletic population that persists with sporting involvement. A retrospective analysis of asymptomatic adolescent athletes identified a progression in spondylolisthesis greater than 5° in 33 out of 86 patients.[89] Although slip progression in the study did not disrupt training or activity participation, another study found that 5 of 20 athletes with symptomatic spondylolisthesis went on to undergo posterolateral fusion for slip progression after initial nonoperative therapy, with 5 more

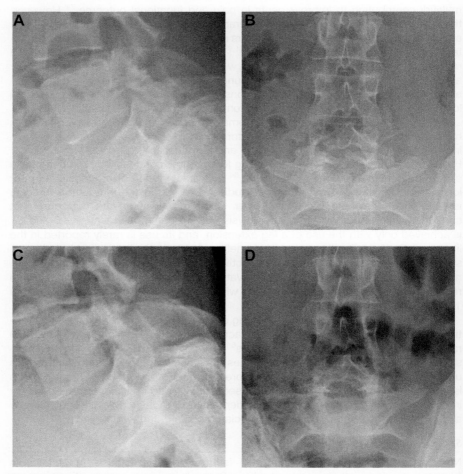

Fig. 3. Lateral and AP radiographs (*A, B*) demonstrating bilateral L5 pars fracture with severe spondylolisthesis of L5 on S1 in a collegiate distance runner. Stable radiographic findings at 2-year follow-up with nonoperative management (*C, D*). AP, anteroposterior.

patients citing persistent pain as their surgical indication.[48] These data suggest that a diagnosis of spondylolisthesis need not dictate a restriction from activity after achieving a pain-free condition from initial therapy. Even though increased deformity is not expected for most patients, a general awareness of the diagnosis may prompt further evaluation in the setting recurrent or persistent pain.

SURGICAL MANAGEMENT

For athletic patients with spondylolysis or low-grade spondylolisthesis, surgical management is typically reserved for those without symptomatic improvement after conservative management for 6 to 12 months. Patients with high-grade spondylolisthesis or significant neurologic deficit may also respond to conservative measures, but many surgeons recommend earlier surgical intervention in these cases. Before surgery, the clinician should exclude other causes of back pain with a thorough history and physical examination and additional diagnostic modalities as indicated. Direct pars fixation and in situ fusion encompass the 2 broad categorizations for the surgical approach to spondylolysis and spondylolisthesis. Although both methods have good postoperative outcomes, direct pars repair obviates surgical extension to adjacent vertebrae, thereby retaining more physiologic mobility, which may be desirable for high-level athletes.

Direct Pars Repair

Direct pars repair involves addressing the direct level of pathology in the lumbar spine. Multiple techniques have been described to stabilize the pars, including Buck compression pedicle screw,[90] Scott wire fixation,[91] and other variations.[92–94] The Buck procedure involves direct visualization with placement of a bone screw across the pars defect, with bony graft placement to promote osseous healing.[90] Multiple studies on the use of Buck procedure in the athletic population demonstrate improvements in functional outcomes with successful return to sport for most patients.[95–100]

Scott's wire fixation technique involves passing a wire through the ipsilateral transverse process and back to the spinous process in a figure-of-8 configuration to compress the pars defect. Nozawa and colleagues[101] studied the Scott wiring technique in athletes, with 18 returning to sport after an extended 12-month rehabilitation process and 3 complications involving the wire construct. Hioki and colleagues[102] correlated improvements in midterm outcome measures by Japanese Orthopedic Association Score with bony union rates on CT, although their study demonstrated nonunion in nearly 20% of their cohort. Debnath and colleagues[95] reported on 22 athletes, with 3 undergoing wire fixation and 19 receiving Buck procedure. Of the patients treated with Scott wiring, one showed no improvement in patient-reported outcome measures and the other two required posterolateral fusion for malunion. Of the patients treated with Buck procedure, 18/19 returned to sport within 7 months with an overall improvement in Short-Form 36 score and Oswestry Disability Index.[95] Although these data suggest that Buck's screw fixation is superior to Scott wiring, there is currently no high-level evidence directly comparing the 2 techniques.

There is also a growing body of literature on the use of minimally invasive approaches for repair of the spondylolysis, although few have reported specifically on athletic patients and outcomes (**Fig. 2**E, F).[103–107] A systematic review comparing minimally invasive surgery to conventional pars repair techniques suggested that patients experienced greater symptomatic improvement in pain, despite an older patient population.[108] With further improvements in surgical technique, tissue-sparing techniques to address spondylolysis may see increased utilization in the near future.

Fusion Techniques

Spinal fusion techniques may be indicated in athletes with spondylolysis and spondylolisthesis. Several variables may be considered when determining the specific method of fixation, including level of pars defect, degree of slippage, and patient-specific considerations. With the L5 pars most commonly injured in isthmic spondylolisthesis, in situ L5-S1 fusion with autogenous posterior iliac graft is commonly used. Extension to L4 may also be indicated with more severe vertebral slippage. Although studies on athletes are limited, studies on in situ fusion in the pediatric population demonstrate good improvement in pain and successful rates of bony union.[109–113] Symptomatic alleviation persists on long-term follow-up of adolescent patients after in situ fusion, without significant degenerative changes in vertebrae proximal to the fixation site.[114,115] Posterolateral fusion is the classic technique described for isthmic spondylolysis, although anterior and circumferential in situ fusion approaches have also shown good functional and radiographic outcomes in high-grade spondylolisthesis (**Fig. 4**).[116]

There is some debate, particularly for the management of severe spondylolisthesis, about the role of vertebral reduction and instrumented fixation. Reduction techniques are potentially advantageous for better cosmetic correction, bony fusion, and sagittal balance.[117] Several nonrandomized retrospective studies have identified improvement in radiographic measures and no difference in short- or midterm clinical outcomes with reduction compared with in situ fusion techniques.[118–120] However, a long-term, retrospective follow-up comparing in situ and reduction found better pain and postoperative function by Scoliosis Research Society scores and lower Oswestry Disability Index scores for the in situ group.[121]

COMPLICATIONS
Iatrogenic Neurologic Deficit

The technical requirements and operative time are increased with reduction and instrumented fixation.[120] The risk of iatrogenic injury has been correlated with the degree of intraoperative reduction for high-grade spondylolisthesis, with particular concern for L5 radiculopathy.[118,122–125] These findings are supported by a frequently cited anatomic study, which showed that a significant portion of L5 nerve strain occurs during the second half of lumbosacral spondylolisthesis reduction.[126] However, the degree of stretch required to incur permanent neurologic deficit is unclear, and investigators variably report the incidence of transient postoperative neuropathy as a complication. It should be noted that a systematic review of retrospective comparative studies on reduction and arthrodesis techniques found no difference in neurologic complications, with overall lower reported rates of neurologic deficit than case series and noncomparative retrospective analyses.[127]

Iatrogenic nerve injury can lead to severe and permanent postoperative deficit without early recognition. In addition to radiculopathy, cauda equina syndrome has been reported with both reduction and in situ techniques.[122,128,129] To minimize the risk of neurologic injury, careful attention should be given to patient positioning or maneuvering, bony decortication, and vertebral reduction. Real-time neurophysiologic monitoring is also recommended. Transient or partial deficits postoperatively may be followed with careful observation. However, for a patient recognized to have significant neurologic deficit, particularly with involvement of bowel and bladder continence, urgent exploration and decompression of nerve roots is indicated.

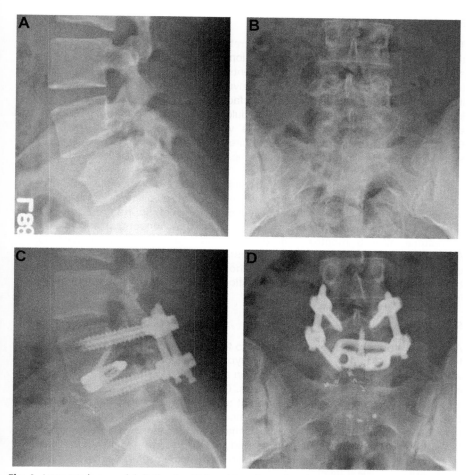

Fig. 4. Low-grade spondylolisthesis of L4 on L5 on lateral and AP radiographs of a collegiate tennis player (A, B). Postoperative imaging 1 year after anterior lumbar interbody fusion and posterior spinal instrumentation and fusion at L4-L5 (C, D).

Pseudoarthrosis

Another complication of surgical correction for spondylolisthesis is the failure of fusion constructs. Pseudarthrosis is seen after various surgical approaches, with high rates reported with in situ fusion techniques.[130,131] A more recent pooled analysis comparing reduction versus in situ fusion found statistically higher rates of pseudoarthrosis in patients undergoing in situ fusion.[127] The risk of pseudoarthrosis is thought to correlate with a high slip angle, although failed fusion does not necessarily correlate with worse clinical outcomes.[132,133] As such, operative intervention should only be considered for those with persistent pain, neurologic symptoms, increasing spinal deformity, or gait disruption.[117]

With such variety of fusion methods described, the risks and benefits of each method should be detailed in the context of patient and family considerations, especially with regard to return to play. Inherent in the risks involved should be a conscious evaluation of the surgeon's prior experience with each surgical technique.

RETURN TO ACTIVITY

The typical signs that patients are safe to return to activity after treatment are alleviation of pain without restricted range of motion, lack of neurologic symptoms or deficits, and stability with activity-specific movements. However, the timeline for return to sport for athletes is variable and depends on a myriad of factors including treatment modality, surgeon-specific protocols, and other factors that motivate recovery such as pre-injury performance and competition schedules. A recent systematic review found that athletes return to sport at 4.3 months with conservative management and at 6.7 months if surgical intervention is required.[134] Some may consider resumption of sport even with symptomatic tolerance if the athlete demonstrates a return to baseline performance.[135]

There are few guidelines addressing the timing for return to contact and noncontact sports after recovery from spondylolysis and spondylolisthesis. Indeed, there is variable consensus among spine surgeons about which sports are appropriate to resume.[136] Generally, most investigators agree that noncontact sports are safe to resume after 6 months with demonstrated recovery and rehabilitation.[137] Although some surgeons believe that patients with spondylolysis should not be participating in contact sports, those who do support a return to contact sports typically recommend a delayed resumption, closer to 12 months after treatment initiation.[136,138–141]

SUMMARY

Athletes are at risk of developing injury to the lumbosacral pars interarticularis due to the repetitive stress exerted during hyperextension, axial loading, and rotation with sporting activity. Pars injury exists on a spectrum from stress reaction to bilateral fracture leading to spondylolisthesis. Clinical evaluation and diagnostic imaging will inform a diagnosis of pars defect and should exclude other causes of low back pain in the athlete. Conservative measures are generally indicated for initial management, and surgical intervention may be considered with persistent symptoms, neurologic deficit, or severe spondylolisthesis. Early identification of injury is important, and many patients return to sport within a year after nonoperative treatment or surgical fixation.

CLINICS CARE POINTS

- Providers should have a high index of suspicion for symptomatic spondylolysis in the athlete presenting with low back pain, regardless of sporting activity.
- Absence of a radiographic "Scotty dog sign" does not exclude injury to the pars interarticularis.
- Consider MRI versus SPECT/CT for initial advanced imaging modality for the evaluation of suspected pars injury.
- Follow-up imaging to demonstrate osseus healing is not necessary for the clinically improving patient but may be warranted with persistent or new-onset pain after initial management.
- Trial of conservative management is appropriate for most athletes presenting with spondylolysis, although early surgical intervention may be considered for severe spondylolisthesis or neurologic deficit.

DISCLOSURE

CC, no funding sources or disclosures. AS, Medtronic: consulting; Nuvasive: consulting and royalties.

REFERENCES

1. Albanese M, Pizzutillo PD. Family study of spondylolysis and spondylolisthesis. J Pediatr Orthop 1982;2(5):496–9.
2. Haukipuro K, Keranen N, Koivisto E, et al. Familial occurrence of lumbar spondylolysis and spondylolisthesis. Clin Genet 1978;13(6):471–6.
3. Wiltse LL. The etiology of spondylolisthesis. J Bone Joint Surg Am 1962;44-A: 539–60.
4. Rosenberg NJ, Bargar WL, Friedman B. The incidence of spondylolysis and spondylolisthesis in nonambulatory patients. Spine (Phila Pa 1976) 1981; 6(1):35–8.
5. Crawford CH 3rd, Ledonio CG, Bess RS, et al. Current evidence regarding the etiology, prevalence, natural history, and prognosis of pediatric lumbar spondylolysis: a report from the scoliosis research society evidence-based medicine committee. Spine Deform 2015;3(1):12–29.
6. Fredrickson BE, Baker D, McHolick WJ, et al. The natural history of spondylolysis and spondylolisthesis. J Bone Joint Surg Am 1984;66(5):699–707.
7. Micheli LJ, Wood R. Back pain in young athletes. Significant differences from adults in causes and patterns. Arch Pediatr Adolesc Med 1995;149(1):15–8.
8. Nitta A, Sakai T, Goda Y, et al. Prevalence of symptomatic lumbar spondylolysis in pediatric patients. Orthopedics 2016;39(3):e434–7.
9. Jackson DW, Wiltse LL, Cirincoine RJ. Spondylolysis in the female gymnast. Clin Orthop Relat Res 1976;117:68–73.
10. Rossi F, Dragoni S. Lumbar spondylolysis: occurrence in competitive athletes. Updated achievements in a series of 390 cases. J Sports Med Phys Fitness 1990;30(4):450–2.
11. Soler T, Calderon C. The prevalence of spondylolysis in the Spanish elite athlete. Am J Sports Med 2000;28(1):57–62.
12. Alvarez-Diaz P, Alentorn-Geli E, Steinbacher G, et al. Conservative treatment of lumbar spondylolysis in young soccer players. Knee Surg Sports Traumatol Arthrosc 2011;19(12):2111–4.
13. Ciullo JV, Jackson DW. Pars interarticularis stress reaction, spondylolysis, and spondylolisthesis in gymnasts. Clin Sports Med 1985;4(1):95–110.
14. Kulling FA, Florianz H, Reepschlager B, et al. High prevalence of disc degeneration and spondylolysis in the lumbar spine of professional beach volleyball players. Orthop J Sports Med 2014;2(4). 2325967114528862.
15. Ruiz-Cotorro A, Balius-Matas R, Estruch-Massana AE, et al. Spondylolysis in young tennis players. Br J Sports Med 2006;40(5):441–6 [discussion 446].
16. Wiltse LL, Newman PH, Macnab I. Classification of spondylolisis and spondylolisthesis. Clin Orthop Relat Res 1976;117:23–9.
17. Marchetti PG, Bartolozzi P. Classification of spondylolisthesis as a guideline for treatment. In: Bridwell KH, DeWald RL, editors. Textbook of spinal surgery. 2nd edition. Philadelphia: Lippincott-Raven; 1997. p. 1211–54.
18. Meyerding HW. Spondylolisthesis. Surg Gynecol Obstet 1932;54:371–7.
19. Herman MJ, Pizzutillo PD. Spondylolysis and spondylolisthesis in the child and adolescent: a new classification. Clin Orthop Relat Res 2005;434:46–54.

20. Mac-Thiong JM, Labelle H. A proposal for a surgical classification of pediatric lumbosacral spondylolisthesis based on current literature. Eur Spine J 2006; 15(10):1425–35.

21. Mac-Thiong JM, Labelle H, Parent S, et al. Reliability and development of a new classification of lumbosacral spondylolisthesis. Scoliosis 2008;3:19.

22. Berger RG, Doyle SM. Spondylolysis 2019 update. Curr Opin Pediatr 2019; 31(1):61–8.

23. Gottlieb LM, Hessler D, Long D, et al. Effects of social needs screening and in-person service navigation on child health: a randomized clinical trial. JAMA Pediatr 2016;170(11):e162521.

24. Fisk JR, Moe JH, Winter RB. Scoliosis, spondylolysis, and spondylolisthesis. Their relationship as reviewed in 539 patients. Spine (Phila Pa 1976) 1978; 3(3):234–45.

25. Sakai T, Goda Y, Tezuka F, et al. Characteristics of lumbar spondylolysis in elementary school age children. Eur Spine J 2016;25(2):602–6.

26. Sakai T, Sairyo K, Takao S, et al. Incidence of lumbar spondylolysis in the general population in Japan based on multidetector computed tomography scans from two thousand subjects. Spine (Phila Pa 1976) 2009;34(21):2346–50.

27. Horn SR, Shepard N, Poorman GW, et al. National trends in the prevalence, treatment, and associated spinal diagnoses among pediatric spondylolysis patients. Bull Hosp Joint Dis 2018;76(4):246–51.

28. Seitsalo S, Osterman K, Poussa M. Scoliosis associated with lumbar spondylolisthesis. A clinical survey of 190 young patients. Spine (Phila Pa 1976) 1988; 13(8):899–904.

29. Jackson DW, Wiltse LL, Dingeman RD, et al. Stress reactions involving the pars interarticularis in young athletes. Am J Sports Med 1981;9(5):304–12.

30. Alqarni AM, Schneiders AG, Cook CE, et al. Clinical tests to diagnose lumbar spondylolysis and spondylolisthesis: a systematic review. Phys Ther Sport 2015;16(3):268–75.

31. Grodahl LH, Fawcett L, Nazareth M, et al. Diagnostic utility of patient history and physical examination data to detect spondylolysis and spondylolisthesis in athletes with low back pain: a systematic review. Man Ther 2016;24:7–17.

32. Sairyo K, Sakai T, Yasui N, et al. Conservative treatment for pediatric lumbar spondylolysis to achieve bone healing using a hard brace: what type and how long? J Neurosurg 2012;16(6):610–4.

33. Millard L. The Scotty dog and his collar. J Ark Med Soc 1976;72(8):339–40.

34. Beck NA, Miller R, Baldwin K, et al. Do oblique views add value in the diagnosis of spondylolysis in adolescents? J Bone Joint Surg Am 2013;95(10):e65.

35. Morimoto M, Sakai T, Goto T, et al. Is the scotty dog sign adequate for diagnosis of fractures in pediatric patients with lumbar spondylolysis? Spine Surg Relat Res 2019;3(1):49–53.

36. Rothman SL, Glenn WV Jr. CT multiplanar reconstruction in 253 cases of lumbar spondylolysis. AJNR Am J Neuroradiol 1984;5(1):81–90.

37. Teplick JG, Laffey PA, Berman A, et al. Diagnosis and evaluation of spondylolisthesis and/or spondylolysis on axial CT. AJNR Am J Neuroradiol 1986;7(3): 479–91.

38. Fadell MF, Gralla J, Bercha I, et al. CT outperforms radiographs at a comparable radiation dose in the assessment for spondylolysis. Pediatr Radiol 2015;45(7): 1026–30.

39. Cheung KK, Dhawan RT, Wilson LF, et al. Pars interarticularis injury in elite athletes - The role of imaging in diagnosis and management. Eur J Radiol 2018; 108:28–42.

40. Dunn AJ, Campbell RSD, Mayor PE, et al. Radiological findings and healing patterns of incomplete stress fractures of the pars interarticularis. Skeletal Radiol 2008;37(5):443–50.

41. Millson HB, Gray J, Stretch RA, et al. Dissociation between back pain and bone stress reaction as measured by CT scan in young cricket fast bowlers. Br J Sports Med 2004;38(5):586–91.

42. Yang JG, Servaes S, Edwards K, et al. Prevalence of stress reaction in the pars interarticularis in pediatric patients with new-onset lower back pain. Clin Nucl Med 2013;38(2):110–4.

43. Bellah RD, Summerville DA, Treves ST, et al. Low-back pain in adolescent athletes: detection of stress injury to the pars interarticularis with SPECT. Radiology 1991;180(2):509–12.

44. Collier BD, Johnson RP, Carrera GF, et al. Painful spondylolysis or spondylolisthesis studied by radiography and single-photon emission computed tomography. Radiology 1985;154(1):207–11.

45. Dutton JA, Hughes SP, Peters AM. SPECT in the management of patients with back pain and spondylolysis. Clin Nucl Med 2000;25(2):93–6.

46. Takemitsu M, El Rassi G, Woratanarat P, et al. Low back pain in pediatric athletes with unilateral tracer uptake at the pars interarticularis on single photon emission computed tomography. Spine 2006;31(8):909–14.

47. Trout AT, Sharp SE, Anton CG, et al. Spondylolysis and beyond: value of SPECT/ CT in evaluation of low back pain in children and young adults. Radiographics 2015;35(3):819–34.

48. Blanda J, Bethem D, Moats W, et al. Defects of pars interarticularis in athletes - a protocol for nonoperative treatment. J Spinal Disord 1993;6(5):406–11.

49. Gregory PL, Batt ME, Kerslake RW, et al. Single photon emission computerized tomography and reverse gantry computerized tomography findings in patients with back pain investigated for spondylolysis. Clin J Sport Med 2005;15(2): 79–86.

50. Gaddikeri S, Matesan M, Alvarez J, et al. MDP-SPECT versus Hybrid MDP-SPECT/CT in the evaluation of suspected pars interarticularis fracture in young athletes. J Neuroimaging 2018;28(6):635–9.

51. Gregory PL, Batt ME, Kerslake RW, et al. The value of combining single photon emission computerised tomography and computerised tomography in the investigation of spondylolysis. Eur Spine J 2004;13(6):503–9.

52. Campbell RSD, Grainger AJ, Hide IG, et al. Juvenile spondylolysis: a comparative analysis of CT, SPECT and MRI. Skeletal Radiol 2005;34(2):63–73.

53. Leone A, Cianfoni A, Cerase A, et al. Lumbar spondylolysis: a review. Skeletal Radiol 2011;40(6):683–700.

54. Kobayashi A, Kobayashi T, Kato K, et al. Diagnosis of radiographically occult lumbar spondylolysis in young athletes by magnetic resonance imaging. Am J Sports Med 2013;41(1):169–76.

55. McCleary MD, Congeni JA. Current concepts in the diagnosis and treatment of spondylolysis in young athletes. Curr Sports Med Rep 2007;6(1):62–6.

56. Alyas F, Turner M, Connell D. MRI findings in the lumbar spines of asymptomatic, adolescent, elite tennis players. Br J Sports Med 2007;41(11):836–41.

57. Jensen MC, Brantzawadzki MN, Obuchowski N, et al. Magnetic-resonance-imaging of the lumbar spine in people without back pain. N Engl J Med 1994; 331(2):69–73.
58. Rajeswaran G, Turner M, Gissane C, et al. MRI findings in the lumbar spines of asymptomatic elite junior tennis players. Skeletal Radiol 2014;43(7):925–32.
59. Ang EC, Robertson AF, Malara FA, et al. Diagnostic accuracy of 3-T magnetic resonance imaging with 3D T1 VIBE versus computer tomography in pars stress fracture of the lumbar spine. Skeletal Radiol 2016;45(11):1533–40.
60. Ganiyusufoglu AK, Onat L, Karatoprak O, et al. Diagnostic accuracy of magnetic resonance imaging versus computed tomography in stress fractures of the lumbar spine. Clin Radiol 2010;65(11):902–7.
61. Hollenberg GM, Beattie PF, Meyers SP, et al. Stress reactions of the lumbar pars interarticularis - The development of a new MRI classification system. Spine 2002;27(2):181–6.
62. Arendt EA, Griffiths HJ. The use of mr imaging in the assessment and clinical management of stress reactions of bone in high-performance athletes. Clin Sports Med 1997;16(2):291–&.
63. Meyers SP, Wiener SN. Magnetic-resonance-imaging features of fractures using the Short Tau Inversion Recovery (Stir) sequence - correlation with radiographic findings. Skeletal Radiol 1991;20(7):499–507.
64. Klein G, Mehlman CT, McCarty M. Nonoperative treatment of spondylolysis and grade I spondylolisthesis in children and young adults: a meta-analysis of observational studies. J Pediatr Orthop 2009;29(2):146–56.
65. Miller SF, Congeni J, Swanson K. Long-term functional and anatomical follow-up of early detected spondylolysis in young athletes. Am J Sports Med 2004;32(4): 928–33.
66. Sys J, Michielsen J, Bracke P, et al. Nonoperative treatment of active spondylolysis in elite athletes with normal X-ray findings: literature review and results of conservative treatment. Eur Spine J 2001;10(6):498–504.
67. Schroeder GD, LaBella CR, Mendoza M, et al. The role of intense athletic activity on structural lumbar abnormalities in adolescent patients with symptomatic low back pain. Eur Spine J 2016;25(9):2842–8.
68. Anderson K, Sarwark JF, Conway JJ, et al. Quantitative assessment with SPECT imaging of stress injuries of the pars interarticularis and response to bracing. J Pediatr Orthop 2000;20(1):28–33.
69. Morita T, Ikata T, Katoh S, et al. Lumbar spondylolysis in children and adolescents. J Bone Joint Surg Br 1995;77(4):620–5.
70. El Rassi G, Takemitsu M, Glutting J, et al. Effect of sports modification on clinical outcome in children and adolescent athletes with symptomatic lumbar spondylolysis. Am J Phys Med Rehabil 2013;92(12):1070–4.
71. Kurd MF, Patel D, Norton R, et al. Nonoperative treatment of symptomatic spondylolysis. J Spinal Disord Tech 2007;20(8):560–4.
72. Nyska M, Constantini N, Cale-Benzoor M, et al. Spondylolysis as a cause of low back pain in swimmers. Int J Sports Med 2000;21(5):375–9.
73. Standaert CJ. Spondylolysis in the adolescent athlete. Clin J Sport Med 2002; 12(2):119–22.
74. O'Sullivan PB, Twomey LT, Allison GT. Evaluation of specific stabilizing exercise in the treatment of chronic low back pain with radiologic diagnosis of spondylolysis or spondylolisthesis. Spine 1997;22(24):2959–67.
75. De Luigi AJ. Low back pain in the adolescent athlete. Phys Med Rehabil Clin N Am 2014;25(4):763–88.

76. Iwamoto J, Takeda T, Wakano K. Returning athletes with severe low back pain and spondylolysis to original sporting activities with conservative treatment. Scand J Med Sci Sports 2004;14(6):346–51.

77. Selhorst M, Fischer A, Graft K, et al. Timing of physical therapy referral in adolescent athletes with acute spondylolysis: a retrospective chart review. Clin J Sport Med 2017;27(3):296–301.

78. Bell DF, Ehrlich MG, Zaleske DJ. Brace treatment for symptomatic spondylolisthesis. Clin Orthop Relat Res 1988;(236):192–8.

79. d'Hemecourt PA, Zurakowski D, Kriemler S, et al. Spondylolysis: returning the athlete to sports participation with brace treatment. Orthopedics 2002;25(6): 653–7.

80. Pizzutillo PD, Hummer CD 3rd. Nonoperative treatment for painful adolescent spondylolysis or spondylolisthesis. J Pediatr Orthop 1989;9(5):538–40.

81. Steiner ME, Micheli LJ. Treatment of symptomatic spondylolysis and spondylolisthesis with the modified Boston brace. Spine (Phila Pa 1976) 1985;10(10): 937–43.

82. Selhorst M, Fischer A, Graft K, et al. Long-term clinical outcomes and factors that predict poor prognosis in athletes after a diagnosis of acute spondylolysis: a retrospective review with telephone follow-up. J Orthop Sport Phys 2016; 46(12):1029–36.

83. Axelsson P, Johnsson R, Stromqvist B. Effect of lumbar orthosis on intervertebral mobility. A roentgen stereophotogrammetric analysis. Spine (Phila Pa 1976) 1992;17(6):678–81.

84. Lantz SA, Schultz AB. Lumbar spine orthosis wearing. II. Effect on trunk muscle myoelectric activity. Spine (Phila Pa 1976) 1986;11(8):838–42.

85. Miller R, Beck NA, Sampson NR, et al. Imaging modalities for low back pain in children: a review of spondyloysis and undiagnosed mechanical back pain. J Pediatr Orthop 2013;33(3):282–8.

86. Danielson BI, Frennered AK, Irstam LK. Radiologic progression of isthmic lumbar spondylolisthesis in young patients. Spine (Phila Pa 1976) 1991;16(4): 422–5.

87. Frennered AK, Danielson BI, Nachemson AL. Natural history of symptomatic isthmic low-grade spondylolisthesis in children and adolescents: a seven-year follow-up study. J Pediatr Orthop 1991;11(2):209–13.

88. Seitsalo S, Osterman K, Hyvarinen H, et al. Progression of spondylolisthesis in children and adolescents. A long-term follow-up of 272 patients. Spine (Phila Pa 1976) 1991;16(4):417–21.

89. Muschik M, Hahnel H, Robinson PN, et al. Competitive sports and the progression of spondylolisthesis. J Pediatr Orthop 1996;16(3):364–9.

90. Buck JE. Direct repair of the defect in spondylolisthesis. Preliminary report. J Bone Joint Surg Br 1970;52(3):432–7.

91. Nicol RO, Scott JH. Lytic spondylolysis. Repair by wiring. Spine (Phila Pa 1976) 1986;11(10):1027–30.

92. Kakiuchi M. Repair of the defect in spondylolysis. Durable fixation with pedicle screws and laminar hooks. J Bone Joint Surg Am 1997;79(6):818–25.

93. Morscher E, Gerber B, Fasel J. Surgical treatment of spondylolisthesis by bone grafting and direct stabilization of spondylolysis by means of a hook screw. Arch Orthop Trauma Surg 1984;103(3):175–8.

94. Sutton JH, Guin PD, Theiss SM. Acute lumbar spondylolysis in intercollegiate athletes. J Spinal Disord Tech 2012;25(8):422–5.

95. Debnath UK, Freeman BJ, Gregory P, et al. Clinical outcome and return to sport after the surgical treatment of spondylolysis in young athletes. J Bone Joint Surg Br 2003;85(2):244–9.

96. Debnath UK, Scammell BE, Freeman BJC, et al. Predictive factors for the outcome of surgical treatment of lumbar spondylolysis in young sporting individuals. Glob Spine J 2018;8(2):121–8.

97. Hardcastle PH. Repair of spondylolysis in young fast bowlers. J Bone Joint Surg Br 1993;75(3):398–402.

98. Menga EN, Kebaish KM, Jain A, et al. Clinical results and functional outcomes after direct intralaminar screw repair of spondylolysis. Spine (Phila Pa 1976) 2014;39(1):104–10.

99. Reitman CA, Esses SI. Direct repair of spondylolytic defects in young competitive athletes. Spine J 2002;2(2):142–4.

100. Roca J, Moretta D, Fuster S, et al. Direct repair of spondylolysis. Clin Orthop Relat Res 1989;(246):86–91.

101. Nozawa S, Shimizu K, Miyamoto K, et al. Repair of pars interarticularis defect by segmental wire fixation in young athletes with spondylolysis. Am J Sports Med 2003;31(3):359–64.

102. Hioki A, Miyamoto K, Sadamasu A, et al. Repair of pars defects by segmental transverse wiring for athletes with symptomatic spondylolysis relationship between bony union and postoperative symptoms. Spine 2012;37(9):802–7.

103. Bartochowski L, Jurasz W, Kruczynski J. A minimal soft tissue damage approach of spondylolysis repair in athletes: preliminary report. Eur J Orthop Surg Traumatol 2017;27(7):1011–7.

104. Gillis CC, Eichholz K, Thoman WJ, et al. A minimally invasive approach to defects of the pars interarticularis: Restoring function in competitive athletes. Clin Neurol Neurosurg 2015;139:29–34.

105. Jin MR, Zhang J, Shao HY, et al. Percutaneous endoscopic-assisted direct repair of pars defect without general anesthesia could be a satisfying treatment alternative for young patient with symptomatic lumbar spondylolysis: a technique note with case series. Bmc Musculoskel Dis 2020;21(1).

106. Zhu X, Wang J, Zhou Y, et al. [Minimally invasive surgery for direct repair of lumbar spondylolysis by utilizing intraoperative navigation and microendoscopic techniques]. Zhongguo Xiu Fu Chong Jian Wai Ke Za Zhi 2015;29(10):1244–8.

107. Nourbakhsh A, Preuss F, Hadeed M, et al. Percutaneous direct repair of a pars defect using intraoperative computed tomography scan: a modification of the buck technique. Spine (Phila Pa 1976) 2017;42(11):E691–4.

108. Kolcun JPG, Chieng LO, Madhavan K, et al. Minimally-invasive versus conventional repair of spondylolysis in athletes: a review of outcomes and return to play. Asian Spine J 2017;11(5):832–42.

109. Helenius I, Lamberg T, Osterman K, et al. Scoliosis research society outcome instrument in evaluation of long-term surgical results in spondylolysis and low-grade isthmic spondylolisthesis in young patients. Spine (Phila Pa 1976) 2005;30(3):336–41.

110. Hensinger RLL, MacEwen G. Surgical management of the spondylolisthesis in children and adolescents. Spine 1976;1:207–15.

111. Jalanko T, Helenius I, Remes V, et al. Operative treatment of isthmic spondylolisthesis in children: a long-term, retrospective comparative study with matched cohorts. Eur Spine J 2011;20(5):766–75.

112. Seitsalo S, Osterman K, Hyvarinen H, et al. Severe spondylolisthesis in children and adolescents. A long-term review of fusion in situ. J Bone Joint Surg Br 1990; 72(2):259–65.
113. Wiltse LL, Jackson DW. Treatment of spondylolisthesis and spondylolysis in children. Clin Orthop Relat Res 1976;117:92–100.
114. Grzegorzewski A, Kumar SJ. In situ posterolateral spine arthrodesis for grades III, IV, and V spondylolisthesis in children and adolescents. J Pediatr Orthop 2000;20(4):506–11.
115. Johnson JR, Kirwan EO. The long-term results of fusion in situ for severe spondylolisthesis. J Bone Joint Surg Br 1983;65(1):43–6.
116. Lamberg T, Remes V, Helenius I, et al. Uninstrumented in situ fusion for high-grade childhood and adolescent isthmic spondylolisthesis: long-term outcome. J Bone Joint Surg Am 2007;89(3):512–8.
117. Cheung EV, Herman MJ, Cavalier R, et al. Spondylolysis and spondylolisthesis in children and adolescents: II. Surgical management. J Am Acad Orthop Surg 2006;14(8):488–98.
118. Molinari RW, Bridwell KH, Lenke LG, et al. Complications in the surgical treatment of pediatric high-grade, isthmic dysplastic spondylolisthesis. A comparison of three surgical approaches. Spine (Phila Pa 1976) 1999;24(16):1701–11.
119. Muschik M, Zippel H, Perka C. Surgical management of severe spondylolisthesis in children and adolescents. Anterior fusion in situ versus anterior spondylodesis with posterior transpedicular instrumentation and reduction. Spine (Phila Pa 1976) 1997;22(17):2036–42 [discussion 2043].
120. Poussa M, Schlenzka D, Seitsalo S, et al. Surgical treatment of severe isthmic spondylolisthesis in adolescents. Reduction or fusion in situ. Spine (Phila Pa 1976) 1993;18(7):894–901.
121. Poussa M, Remes V, Lamberg T, et al. Treatment of severe spondylolisthesis in adolescence with reduction or fusion in situ: long-term clinical, radiologic, and functional outcome. Spine (Phila Pa 1976) 2006;31(5):583–90 [discussion 591-82].
122. DeWald RL, Faut MM, Taddonio RF, et al. Severe lumbosacral spondylolisthesis in adolescents and children. Reduction and staged circumferential fusion. J Bone Joint Surg Am 1981;63(4):619–26.
123. Dick WT, Schnebel B. Severe spondylolisthesis. Reduction and internal fixation. Clin Orthop Relat Res 1988;(232):70–9.
124. Matthiass HH, Heine J. The surgical reduction of spondylolisthesis. Clin Orthop Relat Res 1986;203:34–44.
125. Schar RT, Sutter M, Mannion AF, et al. Outcome of L5 radiculopathy after reduction and instrumented transforaminal lumbar interbody fusion of high-grade L5-S1 isthmic spondylolisthesis and the role of intraoperative neurophysiological monitoring. Eur Spine J 2017;26(3):679–90.
126. Petraco DM, Spivak JM, Cappadona JG, et al. An anatomic evaluation of L5 nerve stretch in spondylolisthesis reduction. Spine (Phila Pa 1976) 1996; 21(10):1133–8 [discussion 1139].
127. Longo UG, Loppini M, Romeo G, et al. Evidence-based surgical management of spondylolisthesis: reduction or arthrodesis in situ. J Bone Joint Surg Am 2014; 96(1):53–8.
128. Burkus JK, Lonstein JE, Winter RB, et al. Long-term evaluation of adolescents treated operatively for spondylolisthesis. A comparison of in situ arthrodesis only with in situ arthrodesis and reduction followed by immobilization in a cast. J Bone Joint Surg Am 1992;74(5):693–704.

129. Schoenecker PL, Cole HO, Herring JA, et al. Cauda equina syndrome after in situ arthrodesis for severe spondylolisthesis at the lumbosacral junction. J Bone Joint Surg Am 1990;72(3):369–77.
130. Boxall D, Bradford DS, Winter RB, et al. Management of severe spondylolisthesis in children and adolescents. J Bone Joint Surg Am 1979;61(4):479–95.
131. Newton PO, Johnston CE 2nd. Analysis and treatment of poor outcomes following in situ arthrodesis in adolescent spondylolisthesis. J Pediatr Orthop 1997;17(6):754–61.
132. Lenke LG, Bridwell KH, Bullis D, et al. Results of in situ fusion for isthmic spondylolisthesis. J Spinal Disord 1992;5(4):433–42.
133. Tsirikos AI, Sud A, McGurk SM. Radiographic and functional outcome of posterolateral lumbosacral fusion for low grade isthmic spondylolisthesis in children and adolescents. Bone Joint J 2016;98-B(1):88–96.
134. Grazina R, Andrade R, Santos FL, et al. Return to play after conservative and surgical treatment in athletes with spondylolysis: a systematic review. Phys Ther Sport 2019;37:34–43.
135. Tallarico RA, Madom IA, Palumbo MA. Spondylolysis and spondylolisthesis in the athlete. Sports Med Arthrosc Rev 2008;16(1):32–8.
136. Rubery PT, Bradford DS. Athletic activity after spine surgery in children and adolescents: results of a survey. Spine (Phila Pa 1976) 2002;27(4):423–7.
137. Standaert CJ, Herring SA. Expert opinion and controversies in sports and musculoskeletal medicine: the diagnosis and treatment of spondylolysis in adolescent athletes. Arch Phys Med Rehabil 2007;88(4):537–40.
138. Bouras T, Korovessis P. Management of spondylolysis and low-grade spondylolisthesis in fine athletes. A comprehensive review. Eur J Orthop Surg Traumatol 2015;25(Suppl 1):S167–75.
139. Burnett MG, Sonntag VK. Return to contact sports after spinal surgery. Neurosurg Focus 2006;21(4):E5.
140. Eck JC, Riley LH 3rd. Return to play after lumbar spine conditions and surgeries. Clin Sports Med 2004;23(3):367–79, viii.
141. Radcliff KE, Kalantar SB, Reitman CA. Surgical management of spondylolysis and spondylolisthesis in athletes: indications and return to play. Curr Sports Med Rep 2009;8(1):35–40.

Axial Low Back Pain in Elite Athletes

Andrew Z. Mo, MD, Joseph P. Gjolaj, MD*

KEYWORDS

- Axial • Low back pain • Athlete • Spondylolysis • Herniation

KEY POINTS

- Lower back pain is prevalent in the general population and in athletes.
- Most patients respond well to conservative treatment.
- A high clinical suspicion and prompt management can prevent worsening or permanent sequelae.

INTRODUCTION

Lower back pain is a common complaint in the general population. An estimated 15% to 20% experience an episode of back pain in a single year. Over the course of a lifetime, 50% to 80% of individuals experience at least 1 episode.[1] Some estimates are higher, estimating the prevalence up to 85% to 95%.[2–4]

Within athletes, back pain is an already complex and vague entity confounded by the specific sport, etiology (traumatic or congenital spine anatomy), and the level of competition of the athlete. Athletic activity in general subjects the body and specifically the spine to extreme physical demand, inducing or exacerbating degenerative changes.[5]

The entirety of the spine is at risk, with catastrophic spinal injuries possible from trauma in higher risk sports such as football, ice hockey, diving, and snowboarding.[6] Axial compression of the spinal column proximally (cervical spine) may lead to fracture and even quadriplegia.[7] In the lumbar spine, sports-associated axial loading forces tend to lead to degenerative changes or disk herniations. There is a direct correlation with increasing lumbar flexion and compressive loads across the intervertebral disk.[8]

Low back pain is more common in athletes of certain sports compared with others. Herniated lumbar disks are most common in football players and weight lifters, degenerative disks and spondylolysis most common in gymnasts, and traumatic lumbar spine injuries most common in wrestlers and hockey players.[9] Sacral fractures are thought to occur more frequently in high-level running sports.[10] In one study of

Department of Orthopaedics, University of Miami Miller School of Medicine, 1120 Northwest 14th Street, 12th Floor, Miami, FL 33136, USA
* Corresponding author.
E-mail address: jgjolaj@miami.edu

Clin Sports Med 40 (2021) 491–499
https://doi.org/10.1016/j.csm.2021.03.005
0278-5919/21/© 2021 Elsevier Inc. All rights reserved.

4790 athletes, 80% of injuries occurred in practice, 6% in competition and 14% in preseason conditioning.[11]

The workup and evaluation of back pain in an athlete requires a careful history, complete neuromuscular examination, and corresponding imaging. The source of the pain can be difficult to identify, secondary to paraspinal musculature, degeneration or herniation of the intervertebral disks, or due to instability from spondylolysis with associated spondylolisthesis. It may also be due to repetitive microtrauma and overuse, leading to acute or chronic injuries such as spondylolysis.[12]

It is often difficult to achieve compliance with nonoperative treatment modalities in the athlete. Although most patients respond clinically positively to cessation of sports, rest, and physical therapy, the competitive nature of athletics often leads to poor compliance. This can result in a deterioration of the condition and ultimately the need for surgical intervention.[3]

The exact source of pain generators may or may not be found. A high index of suspicion and workup is warranted to rule out fractures or soft tissue injuries. Careful history, complete neuromuscular physical examination, and appropriate imaging should be performed.

HISTORY AND PHYSICAL EXAMINATION OF THE ATHLETE

As with all patients who experience spinal pathologies, a detailed history and physical examination are critical in achieving an accurate diagnosis as well as ruling out spine surgical emergencies. Specific questions should include symptom onset, duration, frequency, severity, location of pain, a history of inciting trauma or antecedent injury, and if there is a history of similar pain or symptoms. Red flags or warning signs of night pain, fever, or weight loss should warrant immediate concern for non-musculocutaneous etiologies.

Visual inspection for skin lesions or deformity should be performed, followed by palpation and percussion along the midline and paraspinal musculature. Additional palpation should be performed for possible masses or step off in the posterior element. Other clinical key points to assess for are the presence of pelvic obliquity and leg length discrepancy, gait abnormalities, as well as any deficits or pain in the active range of motion of the lumbar spine. Finally, a complete neurologic examination is critical to assess for motor and sensory function and reflexes.

IMAGING

Plain film radiographs are the first-line diagnostic modality in the evaluation of the athlete with axial low back pain. It is a critical step in the clinical process and should not be skipped in favor of more advanced modalities. Imaging is warranted in the setting of a localized pain or deformity and can both rule out and rule in diagnoses such as spondylolysis, spondylolisthesis, transverse process avulsion fractures, and compression fractures.

Advance imaging modalities are useful in the setting of inconclusive or subtle findings found on plain film. Standard choices are computed tomography (CT) or MRI, with indications and contradictions for both. These are expanded on in further sections. Single photon emission computed tomography may be useful in patients suspected of having spondylolysis.

DIFFERENTIAL

Back pain is a vague symptom, with many descriptors and qualities, but not a true diagnosis. There are many possible etiologies for back pain in the athlete. The most common causes are muscle/ligament strain, degenerative disk disease, disk hernia-tion, isthmic spondylolysis, and isthmic spondylolisthesis (**Box 1**).

Lumbar Strain

Muscular injury typically occurs in the musculotendinous junction, although injury within the muscle belly or insertion can occur as well.[13] Injury occurs to the tissue and muscle fibers without full disruption, and leads to inciting inflammation and pain. Lumbar strains can occur acutely within 48 hours of injury and are associated with muscular spasms. Recurrent muscular strains are characterized by periods without symptoms. Chronic muscle strains are injuries of a greater duration with long-term muscle injury. This category of injury is typically the most found in athletes.[11]

Radiographic workups yield negative results, and on physical examination, findings are nonspecific. The pain may be localized focally to the muscle, or present as a diffuse tightness or dull pain. The diagnosis of lumbar strain is typically of exclusion.

Treatment is nonsurgical, with excellent results and return to play.[14] Rest, icing, and medications are the mainstay of treatment. After a brief period of rest, nonsteroidal anti-inflammatory drugs (NSAIDs), muscle relaxants, and physical therapy should be initiated. The athlete should be pain free with normal function before return to sport.[15–17]

Degenerative Disk Disease

In degenerative disk disease, there are progressive changes that occur with subse-quent disk space narrowing, loss of disk hydration, and altered biomechanics and malalignment. This ultimately leads to abnormal facet loading and eventually facet arthropathy. There has been strong support in the literature for a genetic predisposi-tion for lumbar degenerative changes.[18] It has been suggested in the literature that pa-tients with a first-degree or third-degree relative with degenerative disk disease have a markedly elevated risk.[19] In a study comparing 308 collegiate athletes against a con-trol group of 71 nonathlete university students, there was a considerably higher inci-dence of early lumbar degenerative changes found in the athletic group.[20]

The history and physical examination of patients with degenerative disk disease can also be difficult to elucidate initially. Commonly, a deep, aching lower back pain is

---

Box 1
Differential diagnoses of low back pain

Musculocutaneous in origin
  Muscle strain/sprain
  Muscle contusion
  Degenerative disk disease
  Isthmic spondylolysis
  Isthmic spondylolisthesis
  Disk herniation
  Facet stress fracture
  Sacral stress fracture
  Transverse process avulsion fracture

Other
  Diskitis
  Osteomyelitis
  Neoplasm

described. This pain is worsened by flexion and compressive loads. Relief is achieved with rest and laying in the supine position.

First-line imaging consists of lumbar plain film radiographs to evaluate for abnormal findings including disk space narrowing, subchondral cysts, facet degeneration, and osteophytic changes. Flexion and extension radiographs are helpful in assessing for mobility and stability. CT and MRI provide higher sensitivity and specificity for detecting disk pathology. Hallmark findings include loss of signal intensity on T2-weighted images, annular tears, and associated bone marrow/vertebral end plate changes. It is interesting and important to note that imaging findings do not necessarily correlate with clinical findings: asymptomatic patients may have findings on imaging, or vice versa.[17,21,22]

Lumbar Disk Herniation

Interverbal disks serve an important role in distributing loads and allowing for motion in multiple planes. When a herniation occurs, the inner nucleus pulposus ruptures through the outer annulus, and may cause compression on the nerve roots. Herniations can be classified based on their location (**Fig. 1**). Athletes experience high mechanical stresses during competition and training, and these can include torsional or axial loading of the spine, which may predispose athletes to lumbar disc herniation (LDH).[23] Due to the avascularity of the intervertebral disk, damage is accumulative with limited repair. As noted previously, certain sports, such as weightlifting and football, are at greater risk than others.[9] Sports with repetitive maneuvers can further increase this risk.

When the disk herniates, the nucleus pulposus may be sequestered, extruded, or protruded. The nucleus pulposus can irritate an adjacent nerve root, causing irritation

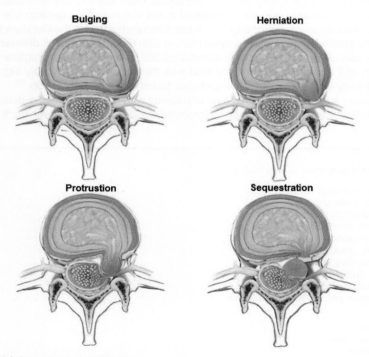

Fig. 1. Disk herniation classifications.

through both mechanical compression and chemical inflammation. Combined, an inflammatory cascade leads to local ischemia, inflammation, and a cascade that leads to radicular pain.

Disk herniations lead to radicular symptoms, often associated with either paresthesia or if severe enough motor weakness. Most disk herniations occur at the L4-5 and L5-S1 levels.[24] Axial back pain and pain in the distribution of sclerotomes are common findings. Additional findings include leg pain, areflexia, and positive leg raise findings. When severe, nerve compression may lead to conus medullaris syndrome or cauda equina syndrome. These surgical emergencies reflect mechanical compression at the level of the spinal cord and cauda equina respectively. Typical presentations include symptoms of severe out-of-proportion leg pain, incontinence, autonomic dysreflexia, and saddle anesthesia. These are clinical diagnoses that require a high index of suspicion and a complete workup including complex imaging such as MRI. Outcomes are improved with surgical decompression within 48 hours.[25] Delays in diagnosis and treatment lead to poor long-term outcomes, with relief of pain but residual bowel and bladder dysfunction.

Radiographs are first line for evaluation and may reveal negative findings. If present, findings include loss of disk height and altered lordosis. CT myelograms and MRI have higher sensitivity and specificity, and will show findings of the disk herniation as well as the affected nerve root to correlate with physical examination findings.[26,27]

Most acute disk herniations will resolve with nonsurgical treatment. MRI observation of patients treated nonsurgically will lead to improvement in more than 90% of patients.[28,29] Sequestered disks have better results of spontaneous resolution and resorption by the body.[30] When nonsurgical treatment fails or in patients with severe motor loss or findings of cauda equina or conus medullaris syndrome, surgical intervention is indicated.

Spondylolysis

Repetitive microtrauma is believed to lead to a defect within the pars interarticularis. This can present either unilaterally or bilaterally and is most commonly observed at the L5-S1 level. With cyclical load, the repetitive trauma leads to fatigue and stress fractures that lead to either elongation or complete fracture and spondylolysis. Young athletes have a higher incidence of symptomatic spondylolysis compared with the general population, with ranges of 15% to 47% compared with 6% to 8%, respectively.[31] This incidence is higher in sports with repetitive extension and loading, such as wrestling, weight lifting, and diving.[32] The prevalence of spondylolysis has been reported to be as high as 38% and 44% in professional soccer and baseball players, respectively.[33] Spondylolisthesis can subsequently follow in the setting of bilateral spondylolysis, with anterior-posterior displacement of adjacent vertebral bodies. This is classified according to the Meyerding classification (**Table 1**).[34]

Typically, there is a mechanical midline lower back pain or focal unilateral symptoms in the setting of a unilateral pars defect. With no listhesis present, the pain is typically localized and exacerbated by repetitive activities that include hyperextension of the lumbar spine. When spondylolisthesis is present, neurologic symptoms, primarily L5 radiculopathy due to L5-S1 being the most common, will result from foraminal stenosis.

Patients are diagnosed with a careful history, examination, and reviewing of imaging. Upright lateral lumbar radiographs are first line and may show listhesis if present with severe bilateral pars defects. On an oblique lumbar radiograph, a pathognomonic "Scottie dog sign" will result from a radiolucency through the pars interarticularis

Table 1
Meyerding classification of spondylolisthesis

Grade	Ratio[a]
I	0%–25%
II	25%–50%
III	50%–75%
IV	75%–100%
V	>100%

[a] Percent listhesis of superior to inferior vertebral body.

(**Fig. 2**). CT imaging is more sensitive but used judiciously due to the additional radiation exposure.[35]

Although due to a physical defect, either unilaterally or bilaterally in the pars intraarticularis, most athletes will respond positively to conservative treatment. After a brief period of rest, on the order of several days, physical rehabilitation, NSAIDs and bracing are used. Patients will typically either heal with bony union or a fibrous nonunion, but if asymptomatic they may be observed and return to play.[36–39]

In the event of continued pain despite nonsurgical interventions, surgical treatment is indicated. Indications include neurologic deficit related to nerve root compromise, intractable pain, and poor alignment clinically. Surgical options include a direct posterolateral fusion and direct pars repair, whether performed through a traditional open or more contemporary minimally invasive approach.

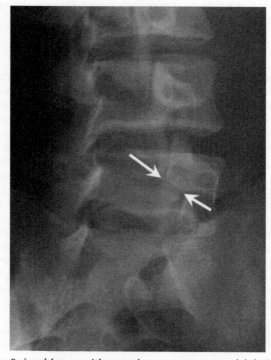

Fig. 2. "Scottie Dog" sign (shown with *arrow*) represents a spondylolysis or fracture of the pars intraarticularis and is visible on the oblique radiographic view of the lumbar spine.

SUMMARY

Low back pain is a common symptom resulting from various etiology. It is prevalent almost universally in the general population and within competitive athletes. Although varying in causation and severity, most commonly transient and mechanical in nature, a high index of suspicion and a thorough history and physical are paramount to rule out rarer causes that may be associated with potentially devastating sequela. Most symptoms can be treated with nonsurgical care, including but not limited to rest, cessation of activity, NSAIDs, and physical therapy. In situations of refractory or progressing symptoms, surgical management should be considered as necessary. A team approach involving the coach, athlete, and physician can help to identify and treat pain generators and minimize long-term injury.

CLINICS CARE POINTS

- Low back pain is highly prevalent in the general population and in athletes.
- Most patients respond well to conservative treatment.
- Red flag signs of fever, weight loss, and night pain should warrant workup for non-musculocutaneous causes.
- A high clinical suspicion and prompt management can prevent worsening or permanent sequelae.

DISCLOSURE

J.P. Gjolaj- Depuy-Synthes (consulting), NuVasive (consulting, research support). A.Z. Mo - None.

REFERENCES

1. Rubin DI. Epidemiology and risk factors for spine pain. Neurol Clin 2007;25(2): 353–71.
2. Wang MY, Berven SH. Lumbar pedicle subtraction osteotomy. Neurosurgery 2007;60(2 SUPPL.1):140–6.
3. Lawrence JP, Greene HS, Grauer JN. Back pain in athletes. J Am Acad Orthop Surg 2006;14(13):726–35.
4. Trainor TJ, Wiesel SW. Epidemiology of back pain in the athlete. Clin Sports Med 2002;21(1):93–103.
5. Cholewicki J, McGill SM, Norman RW. Lumbar spine loads during the lifting of extremely heavy weights. Med Sci Sports Exerc 1991;23(10):1179–86.
6. Boden BP, Tacchetti RL, Cantu RC, et al. Catastrophic head injuries in high school and college football players. Am J Sports Med 2007;35(7):1075–81.
7. Boden BP, Jarvis CG. Spinal Injuries in Sports. Neurol Clin 2008;26(1):63–78.
8. Cappozzo A, Felici F, Figura F, et al. Lumbar spine loading during half-squat exercises. Med Sci Sports Exerc 1985;17(5):613–20.
9. Gerbino PG, d'Hemecourt PA. Does football cause an increase in degenerative disease of the lumbar spine? Curr Sports Med Rep 2002;1(1):47–51.
10. Bono CM. Current Concepts Review: Low-Back Pain in Athletes. J Bone Joint Surg Am 2004;86(2):382–96.
11. Keene JS, Albert MJ, Springer SL, et al. Back injuries in college athletes. J Spinal Disord 1989;2(3):190–5.

12. Morita T, Ikata T, Katoh S, et al. Lumbar spondylolysis in children and adolescents. J Bone Joint Surg Br 1995;77(4):620–5.

13. Keene JS, Drummond DS. Mechanical back pain in the athlete. Compr Ther 1985;11(1):7–14.

14. Haus BM, Micheli LJ. Back Pain in the Pediatric and Adolescent Athlete. Clin Sports Med 2012;31(3):423–40.

15. Dreisinger TE, Nelson B. Management of back pain in athletes. Sport Med 1996; 21(4):313–20.

16. Young JL, Press JM, Herring SA. The disc at risk in athletes: perspectives on operative and nonoperative care. Med Sci Sports Exerc 1997;29(7 SUPPL). https://doi.org/10.1097/00005768-199707001-00004.

17. Boden SD, Davis DO, Dina TS, et al. Abnormal magnetic-resonance scans of the lumbar spine in asymptomatic subjects. A prospective investigation. J Bone Joint Surg Am 1990;72(3):403–8.

18. Battié MC, Videman T, Kaprio J, et al. The Twin Spine Study: Contributions to a changing view of disc degeneration†. Spine J 2009;9(1):47–59.

19. Hsu WK, Jenkins TJ. Management of lumbar conditions in the elite athlete. J Am Acad Orthop Surg 2017;25(7):489–98.

20. Hangai M, Kaneoka K, Hinotsu S, et al. Lumbar intervertebral disk degeneration in athletes. Am J Sports Med 2009;37(1):149–55.

21. Borenstein DG, O'Mara J, Boden SD, et al. The value of magnetic resonance imaging of the lumbar spine to predict low-back pain in asymptomatic subjects: A seven-year follow-up study. J Bone Joint Surg Am 2001;83(9):1306–11.

22. Boden SD, Davis DO, Dina TS, et al. Abnormal magnetic-resonance scans of the lumbar spine in asymptomatic subjects. A prospective investigation. J Bone Joint Surg Am 1990;72(3):403–8.

23. Hsu WK, McCarthy KJ, Savage JW, et al. The Professional Athlete Spine Initiative: outcomes after lumbar disc herniation in 342 elite professional athletes. Spine J 2011;11(3):180–6.

24. Weinstein JN, Lurie JD, Tosteson TD, et al. Surgical versus nonoperative treatment for lumbar disc herniation. Spine (Phila Pa 1976) 2008;33(25):2789–800.

25. Ahn UM, Ahn NU, Buchowski JM, et al. Cauda equina syndrome secondary to lumbar disc herniation. Spine (Phila Pa 1976) 2000;25(12):1515–22.

26. Maravilla KR, Lesh P, Weinreb JC, et al. Magnetic resonance imaging of the lumbar spine with CT correlation. AJNR Am J Neuroradiol 1985;6(2):237–45.

27. Jackson RP, Cain JE, Jacobs RR, et al. The neuroradiographic diagnosis of lumbar herniated nucleus pulposus: II. A comparison of computed tomography (CT), myelography, CT-myelography, and magnetic resonance imaging. Spine (Phila Pa 1976) 1989;14(12):1362–7.

28. Cribb GL, Jaffray DC, Cassar-Pullicino VN. Observations on the natural history of massive lumbar disc herniation. J Bone Joint Surg Br 2007;89(6):782–4.

29. Bozzao A, Gallucci M, Masciocchi C, et al. Lumbar disk herniation: MR imaging assessment of natural history in patients treated without surgery. Radiology 1992; 185:135–41.

30. Macki M, Hernandez-Hermann M, Bydon M, et al. Spontaneous regression of sequestrated lumbar disc herniations: literature review. Clin Neurol Neurosurg 2014; 120:136–41.

31. Brooks BK, Southam SL, Mlady GW, et al. Lumbar spine spondylolysis in the adult population: using computed tomography to evaluate the possibility of adult onset lumbar spondylosis as a cause of back pain. Skeletal Radiol 2010;39(7):669–73.

32. Rossi F, Dragoni S. Lumbar spondylolysis: occurrence in competitive athletes. Updated achievements in a series of 390 cases. J Sports Med Phys Fitness 1990;30(4):450–2.
33. Sakai T, Sairyo K, Suzue N, et al. Incidence and etiology of lumbar spondylolysis: review of the literature. J Orthop Sci 2010;15(3):281–8.
34. Meyerding H. Spondylolisthesis. Surg Gynecol Obs 1932;(54):371–7.
35. Campbell RSD, Grainger AJ, Hide IG, et al. Juvenile spondylolysis: a comparative analysis of CT, SPECT and MRI. Skeletal Radiol 2005;34(2):63–73.
36. Jackson DW, Wiltse LL, Dingeman RD, et al. Stress reactions involving the pars interarticularis in young athletes. Am J Sports Med 1981;9(5):304–12.
37. Blanda J, Bethem D, Moats W, et al. Defects of pars interarticularis in athletes: a protocol for nonoperative treatment. J Spinal Disord 1993;6(5):406–11.
38. Steiner ME, Micheli LJ. Treatment of symptomatic spondylolysis and spondylolisthesis with the modified Boston brace. Spine (Phila Pa 1976) 1985;10(10): 937–43.
39. Sys J, Michielsen J, Bracke P, et al. Nonoperative treatment of active spondylolysis in elite athletes with normal X-ray findings: literature review and results of conservative treatment. Eur Spine J 2001;10(6):498–504.

Lumbar Disk Herniations and Radiculopathy in Athletes

Paul R. Gause, MD*, Ryan J. Godinsky, MD, Keven S. Burns, MD, Edward J. Dohring, MD

KEYWORDS

- Athlete • Lumbar disk herniation • Lumbar disc herniation • Radiculopathy
- Microdiskectomy

KEY POINTS

- Lumbar disk herniation (LDH) is a common cause of morbidity in athletes with low back pain.
- Underlying degenerative disk disease is prevalent in athletes and is a risk factor for the development of LDH.
- Given the pressures regarding return to play, athletes are more likely to undergo surgical intervention earlier in their treatment course.
- Return to play after LDH is favorable; however, career duration and return to preinjury performance level may be affected.

INTRODUCTION

Lumbar disk herniation (LDH) is a common cause of morbidity and health care cost in the United States. It is estimated 2% of the population will suffer from a symptomatic LDH in their lifetime.[1] Given the physical demands placed across the lumbar spine in various sports, athletes are known to have a higher lifetime incidence of low back pain (LBP) compared with the general public.[2] Although the main causes of LBP in athletes are musculoligamentous strain, degenerative disk disease (DDD), and spondylolysis, it is has been reported that up to 11% of acute cases of LBP are a result of LDH.[3,4]

To alleviate symptomatology and facilitate return to sport, a thorough understanding of the pathoanatomy, clinical presentation, diagnosis, and treatment of LDH is paramount.

PATHOANATOMY

The intervertebral disk is composed of a central nucleus pulposus (NP) and an outer fibrous ring known as the annulus fibrosus (AF). The central NP is composed of type

Spine Institute of Arizona, 9735 North 90th Place, Scottsdale, AZ 85258, USA
* Corresponding author.
E-mail address: PaulG@SpineAZ.com

Clin Sports Med 40 (2021) 501–511
https://doi.org/10.1016/j.csm.2021.04.001
0278-5919/21/© 2021 Elsevier Inc. All rights reserved.

Il collagen and contains proteoglycans that bind water molecules. The high water content of the NP and resultant hydrostatic pressure functions to resist axial compression of the spine. In comparison, the AF is composed of primarily type I collagen and contains far fewer proteoglycans and thus fewer water molecules. The AF serves as a tensile ring that contains the NP and serves as an attachment to the corresponding vertebral body endplates. When the intervertebral disk is placed under axial load, the NP flattens and generates a tensile hoop stress. The AF functions to resist this generated force. Formation of an LDH occurs when this generated force disrupts a portion or the entire thickness of the AF and it no longer appropriately contains the NP.[5]

Force generation across a healthy intervertebral disk is well established in the literature. When standing upright, an individual generates 440 Newtons (N) across a lumbar motion segment. This force increases to 1190 N when one remains upright and forward flexes at the waist. Sitting in a relaxed position generates 380 N, whereas bending forward increases the force to 1130 N.[6] A previous cadaveric study demonstrated failure of the AF and formation of a disk protrusion when an average force of 5448 N was applied with a flexion angle of 12.8° across the lumbar intervertebral disk (IVD).[7]

Although athletes are typically better conditioned than the general public, the demands of sport often place the lumbar spine under significant loads. Gatt and colleagues[8] investigated the forces generated across the L4-5 disk in Division I-A college football linemen. They reported an average force generation of 8679 N during a typical blocking sequence. An analysis of professional and amateur golfers concluded that 7500 N and 6100 N of force are generated across the L3-4 motion segment, respectively.[9] Cholewicki and colleagues[10] studied world-class power lifters and noted an average compressive load of 17,192 N acting across the L4-5 motion segment during dead lifts. The work of Hosea and Hannafin[11] with elite rowers documented an average cyclical load of 6100 N. The demands athletes place across their lumbar spines is likely a predisposing factor in the development of lumbar pathology.

PREDISPOSING FACTORS

The natural aging process leads to biochemical and biomechanical changes within the intervertebral disk. Loss of proteoglycans within the NP leads to decreased water content and disk desiccation. In addition, degradation of the extracellular matrix and changes in local pH further contribute to this process. Progressive loss of NP size, pressurization, and disk height alter the normal load-bearing characteristics of the IVD. The altered NP can no longer handle compressive forces as effectively, leading to increased force transmission across the AF and the propensity for disruption.[12]

Various genetic factors have been studied and linked to DDD and early desiccation. It is believed that up to 75% of early DDD is a result of genetic predisposition. Genes regulating collagen formation, matrix metalloproteinases, structural proteins, and various growth factors, as well as apoptosis-regulating genes have all been implicated in this phenomenon.[13]

Preexisting DDD has been linked to an increased incidence of LDH.[14] A high prevalence of DDD has been reported in various sports. In 1991, Swärd and colleagues[15] reported DDD in 75% of elite male gymnasts with an average age of 18, versus 31% in age-matched controls. A study conducted at the 2016 Olympic Summer Games in Rio de Janeiro found 39% of screened athletes had preexisting lumbar DDD. The investigators concluded that in comparison with previously reported age-matched controls, these athletes had higher rates of moderate to severe degenerative changes.[16]

Multiple studies have reported a high prevalence of DDD in football linemen.[17] Rajeswaran and colleagues[18] evaluated 98 asymptomatic junior elite tennis players and found that 62% had underlying DDD. A study of 75 elite alpine skiers, age range 16 to 20 years, found a prevalence of DDD in 56% of those studied versus 30% in age-matched controls.[19] The high prevalence of DDD among athletes may place them at increased risk for development of LDH.

SIGNS, SYMPTOMS, PHYSICAL EXAMINATION, AND DIAGNOSTIC GUIDELINES

Symptoms associated with LDH include axial LBP, radicular pain, and possible sensorimotor deficits. Symptoms vary depending on the size, location, and inflammatory response of the LDH. After the inciting event, it is not uncommon for the patient to experience a prodrome of LBP followed by dysesthesias, paresthesias, and/or numbness. Patients may exhibit motor dysfunction in a specific lumbosacral nerve root. Central LDHs typically present with axial back pain without radicular features, whereas paracentral LDHs are more likely to have radicular features, given their proximity to the traversing nerve root. Severe cases of LDH can present as cauda equina syndrome (CES). CES represents a constellation of motor and sensory disturbances of the lower extremities coupled with saddle anesthesia, and potential bladder, bowel, and/or sexual dysfunction.

Symptoms of LDH may be exacerbated by straining, coughing, and sneezing, as these actions lead to increased intrathecal pressure. Forward flexion at the waist and sitting load the anterior column and increase the intradiskal pressure by up to 40%.[20] Clinical signs associated with LDH include the straight leg raise, contralateral straight leg raise, and the femoral stretch test. These examinations stretch an already irritated nerve root and may lead to increase in radicular complaints.

The sensory and motor findings vary based on the level and location of the disk herniation. Ninety-five percent of LDHs occur at L4/5 and L5/S1. Between 95% and 98% of LDHs are described as central or paracentral in nature. Paracentral is the most common location, as it is just lateral to the lateral boundaries of the posterior longitudinal ligament. Paracentral LDHs occur near the traversing nerve root (**Fig. 1**). As a result, a paracentral LDH at L4/5 often manifests with L5 radicular symptoms. In comparison, a far-lateral LDH (**Fig. 2**), which is much less common, will affect the exiting nerve root (L4 root at the L4/5 level).[21,22]

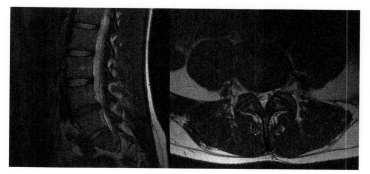

Fig. 1. Right paracentral disk herniation at L4/5 in an 18-year-old athlete. Sagittal (*left*) and axial (*right*) T2-weighted MRI images. Patient had right buttock, posterolateral thigh, and lateral leg pain in a classic L5 distribution.

The North American Spine Society's Evidence-Based Guideline Development Committee recommends manual muscle testing, sensory testing, and classic and crossed straight leg raise as the gold standard for clinical diagnosis of LDH (grade of recommendation: A).[23] Rabin and colleagues[24] found that there is a statistical difference in favor of the supine straight leg raise over the seated straight leg raise with the sensitivity of 0.67 versus 0.41, respectively. They found insufficient evidence to make a recommendation for or against the use of the cough impulse test, Bell test, hyperextension test, femoral nerve stretch test, slump test, lumbar range of motion, or absence of reflexes in diagnosing LDH with radiculopathy (grade of recommendation: I).[24]

IMAGING
Radiographs

Lumbar radiographs are the first-line imaging modality used in evaluating LBP with or without radiculopathy. In the absence of red flags, radiographs are indicated after completing 6 weeks of conservative care. Weight-bearing anteroposterior and lateral radiographs assess overall alignment, presence of transitional anatomy, DDD, spondylosis, spondylolisthesis, and fracture. It is the authors' recommendation to include flexion and extension radiographs to evaluate for underlying instability. Potential radiographic findings of LDH include compensatory scoliosis and endplate avulsion fracture.

MRI

MRI is the gold standard for confirmation of a suspected LDH. MRI has the highest sensitivity and specificity among imaging modalities for the confirmation of LDH.[25] When recurrent LDH is suspected, intravenous gadolinium contrast can be used to delineate LDH from epidural fibrosis.

Computed Tomography

Given the diagnostic accuracy of MRI, the role of computed tomography (CT) is limited to individuals who have a contraindication to MRI. Previous studies have compared CT alone versus CT myelogram in the diagnosis of LDH. Myelogram increases the sensitivity and specificity of CT.[25] If MRI is contraindicated, a post myelogram CT is recommended.

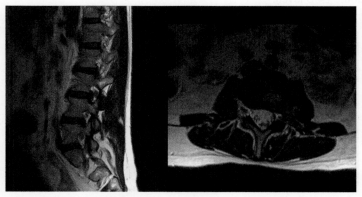

Fig. 2. Left foraminal (far-lateral) disk herniation at L3/4 in a 32-year-old woman. Sagittal (*left*) and axial (*right*) T2-weighted MRI images. Patient had left buttock, lateral hip, and anterior thigh pain in a classic L3 distribution.

Treatment

Although the general treatment algorithm of athletes with LDH is similar to nonathletes, sport-specific factors are often considered. The timing of one's injury with respect to the season, the demands of the sport, and contractual and monetary factors influence the decision-making process. Although the mainstay of treatment of symptomatic LDH is multimodal conservative care, elite athletes are more likely to undergo surgical intervention.[26]

NONOPERATIVE TREATMENT

Nonsurgical care, including pain management and functional restoration, is the mainstay of initial treatment. As in the nonathletic population, nonsurgical care is associated with a high chance of success and return to play in the athletic population.[27] Previous literature has documented that 90% of patients with a known symptomatic LDH have favorable outcomes with conservative care.[28] Initial care consists of a short period of rest to last no more than 1 week followed by early mobilization and the initiation of formal physical therapy.[29] Physical therapy focuses on core stability and strengthening, lower extremity flexibility, and maintaining truncal and lower extremity mobility. Given the high level of physical conditioning in athletes before their injury state, earlier and more rigorous therapy is often initiated. In addition, elite athletes have access to state-of-the-art training facilities and providers to guide and tailor their therapy protocols.[30]

Oral pharmacologic therapy is also considered a first-line treatment for symptomatic LDH. Nonsteroidal anti-inflammatory drugs (NSAIDs) decrease inflammatory cytokine mediator production by inhibiting cyclooxygenase enzyme function. NSAIDs have shown a small treatment effect in symptomatic LDH.[31] Corticosteroids also decrease inflammatory cytokine production by downregulating gene expression associated with cytokine production. A randomized clinical trial examining the use of corticosteroids in symptomatic LDH showed a modest improvement in function, but no reduction in pain at 3 weeks.[32] Gabapentinoids (gabapentin, pregabalin), which bind voltage-dependent calcium channels, are frequently used in neuropathic pain.[33] Although these medications are commonly used for lumbar radicular pain resulting from LDH, studies have shown them to be ineffective.[34] Muscle relaxants, a diverse group of medications that can be classified into antispasmodics and antispastics, work by altering central nervous system conduction or directly improving muscle tonicity and spasm directly through the spinal cord or skeletal muscle, respectively. Limited data are available on the use of muscle relaxants and their efficacy in treating LDH.[35]

Lumbar epidural steroid injections (ESIs), including interlaminar and transforaminal, are commonly used as second-line agents in the treatment of symptomatic LDH. The literature is contradictory regarding the efficacy of injection therapy. ESIs have been shown to be effective in reducing pain and radicular symptoms in 20% to 85% of those with a symptomatic acute LDH.[36,37] Their mechanism of action is to decrease the local inflammatory cascade and stabilization of the nerve cell membrane. Thus, the role of ESI is best suited in the inflammatory stage and for the reduction of acute pain and dysfunction. Multiple studies have shown that ESIs do not reduce the potential need for surgery.[38]

Evaluating conservative care versus surgical intervention in athletes, Iwamoto and colleagues[39] compared 1 prospective and 6 retrospective studies of symptomatic LDH. The investigators found no difference in return to play in athletes treated operatively versus nonoperatively. Of those treated conservatively, they reported a return to play of 78.9% at an average of 4.7 months.[39]

OPERATIVE TREATMENT

In the absence of red flags (acute/progressive motor deficit, loss of bowel or bladder function), surgical candidates for LDH are those who have failed nonoperative management over a course of at least 6 weeks. In the elite athlete, relative indications for surgery include inability to perform their sport after a course of conservative care. The timeline of conservative care may be different in the athlete population given the multitude of variables associated with their return to play and their level of conditioning. Typically, surgery is considered earlier with elite athletes than the general population.

The standard operative treatment for LDH is a laminotomy with diskectomy. Multiple surgical techniques have been described, including traditional open laminotomy with diskectomy, minimally invasive tubular microdiskectomy (**Fig. 3**), and endoscopic microdiskectomy. Multiple large studies have shown that operative management of LDH improves short-term outcomes; however, the difference is controversial at mid-range and long-range outcomes when compared with conservative care.[40,41]

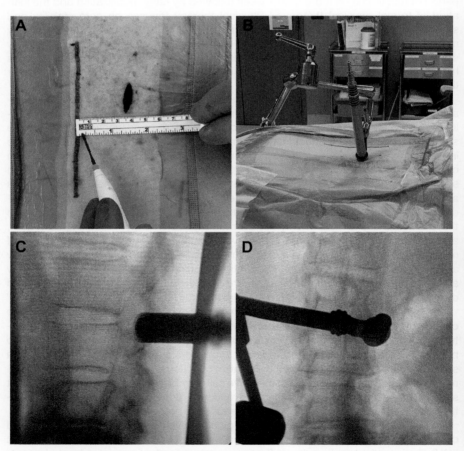

Fig. 3. Far-lateral microdiskectomy. Incision placed 4 cm lateral to midline (*A*). Dilators placed to allow placement of tubular retractor (*B*). AP and lateral fluoroscopic views with tubular retractor docked at the superior aspect of the transverse process (*C,D*).

Over the past 2 decades, the use of minimally invasive spine surgery has become more common. Advantages of tubular and endoscopic microdiskectomy over a traditional open approach have been established. Minimally invasive techniques provide adequate visualization of the operative field through a smaller skin incision, thus creating less disturbance of the surrounding anatomy. Literature has shown lower rates of infection, decreased blood loss, less injury to the lumbar paraspinals, as well as decreased postoperative pain in those undergoing minimally invasive microdiskectomy (tubular and endoscopic). Minimally invasive techniques do have a higher rate of certain complications, including incomplete decompression, residual radicular pain, incidental durotomy, and reherniation. Previous studies attribute the increased complication rate to the steep learning curve associated with minimally invasive techniques.[42,43]

Matsunga and colleagues[44] reported that 81% of athletes who underwent endoscopic microdiskectomy returned to play. They noted that those athletes who returned to play did so at an average of 2 months; this was faster than any other technique. Regardless of surgical technique, outcomes following surgical intervention are favorable. A 2015 metanalysis containing 39,048 patients who underwent surgical intervention for symptomatic LDH reported 79% had good/excellent outcomes at a follow-up of 2.9 to 6.3 years.[45] In addition, the 8-year data from the Spine Patient Outcome Research Trial (SPORT) showed a reoperation rate of 14.7% for those treated initially with microdiskectomy, which was less than previously published data.[46] Like any surgery, there are potential complications with surgical intervention. Commonly reported complications in the treatment of symptomatic LDH include infection, durotomy, and reherniation.

RETURN TO PLAY

The Professional Athlete Spine Initiative reported on the outcome of 342 elite athletes from the 4 major North American sports who underwent treatment of a symptomatic LDH. Hsu and colleagues[26] reported a return to play in 82% of athletes, with an average postinjury length of career of 3.4 years; 226 of the athletes underwent surgical intervention, whereas 116 underwent conservative care. There was no difference in return to play or career length between the surgical and nonsurgical cohorts. The investigators reported the highest return to play in Major League Baseball and the lowest in the National Football League.[26] Watkins and colleagues[47] reported work with professional and Olympic athletes who underwent lumbar microdiskectomy for symptomatic LDH. The findings were similar, reporting a return to play of 88% at an average of 5.2 months from time of intervention.[47] In a study of 61 National Basketball Association players with symptomatic LDH, of whom 34 underwent microdiskectomy and 27 were treated nonoperatively, return to play was 77.8% in the nonoperative group and 79.4% in the operative group. The investigators found that the operative group played more postinjury seasons that the nonoperative group.[48] Weistroffer and Hsu[49] reported on a series of 66 NFL linemen with symptomatic LDH. In their series, 52 were treated surgically and 14 conservatively; 80.8% (42 of 52) returned to play in the surgical cohort whereas only 28.6% (4 of 14) returned to play in those treated nonsurgically. Of those who returned to play from the surgical cohort, their average length of career after return was 3 years, with 33 games played on average.[49,50] Last, a study of 87 National Hockey League players with symptomatic LDH showed an average return to play of 85% regardless of intervention. There was not a difference noted in return to play between surgical and nonsurgical cohorts. The investigators noted average games played dropped from 56.2 preinjury to 39 postinjury. In addition, performance declined from 0.22 point per game (ppg) to 0.17 ppg postinjury.

SUMMARY

LBP and lumbar pathology are common findings in athletes. The incidence of LDH in athletes with LBP has been reported as high as 11%. Previous studies have shown underlying DDD as a preexisting risk factor for those who develop an LDH. Multiple studies have reported an increased prevalence of DDD in elite athletes across multiple sports. Although most patients who develop a symptomatic LDH improve with conservative care, athletes pose a more difficult treatment algorithm. The pressure to return to sport at their preinjury performance level often influences the type of intervention and its timing. Current literature supports favorable return to sport after symptomatic LDH. Although operative intervention may result in faster return to play, no significant differences have been reported in the literature. Given the unique demands of each sport, a patient-specific and sport-specific treatment algorithm is necessary for maximize return to play and its duration.

CLINICS CARE POINTS

- Nonoperative care of symptomatic LDH is associated with favorable outcomes across all populations, including athletes.
- The timeline of conservative care may be different in the athlete population given the multitude of variables associated with their return to play and their pre-injury level of conditioning.
- Although operative intervention may result in faster return to play, no significant differences have been reported comparing non-operative versus operative intervention in symptomatic lumbar disk herniation.
- Given the unique demands of each sport, a patient-specific and sport-specific treatment algorithm is necessary for maximize return to play and its duration.

DISCLOSURE

The authors have nothing to disclose.

REFERENCES

1. Fatoye F, Gebrye T, Odeyemi I. Real-world incidence and prevalence of low back pain using routinely collected data. Rheumatol Int 2019;39(4):619–26.
2. Trompeter K, Fett D, Platen P. Prevalence of back pain in sports: a systematic review of the literature. Sports Med 2017;47(6):1183–207.
3. Mortazavi J, Zebardast J, Mirzashahi B. Low back pain in athletes. Asian J Sports Med 2015;6(2):e24718.
4. Micheli LJ, Wood R. Back pain in young athletes. Significant differences from adults in causes and patterns. Arch Pediatr Adolesc Med 1995;149(1):15–8.
5. Walker MH, Anderson DG. Molecular basis of intervertebral disc degeneration. Spine J 2004;4(6 Suppl):158S–66S.
6. Schultz A, Andersson G, Ortengren R, et al. Loads on the lumbar spine. Validation of a biomechanical analysis by measurements of intradiscal pressures and myoelectric signals. J Bone Joint Surg Am 1982;64(5):713–20.
7. Adams MA, Hutton WC. Prolapsed intervertebral disc. A hyperflexion injury 1981 Volvo Award in Basic Science. Spine (Phila Pa 1976) 1982;7(3):184–91.

8. Gatt CJ Jr, Hosea TM, Palumbo RC, et al. Impact loading of the lumbar spine during football blocking. Am J Sports Med 1997;25(3):317–21.

9. Hosea TM, Gatt CJ, McCarthy KE, et al. Analytic computation of rapid dynamic loading of the lumbar spine. Trans Orthop Res Soc 1989;14:358.

10. Cholewicki J, McGill SM, Norman RW. Lumbar spine loads during the lifting of extremely heavy weights. Med Sci Sports Exerc 1991;23(10):1179–86.

11. Hosea TM, Hannafin JA. Rowing injuries. Sports Health 2012;4(3):236–45.

12. Vo NV, Hartman RA, Patil PR, et al. Molecular mechanisms of biological aging in intervertebral discs. J Orthop Res 2016;34(8):1289–306.

13. Martirosyan NL, Patel AA, Carotenuto A, et al. Genetic alterations in intervertebral disc disease. Front Surg 2016;3:59.

14. Raudner M, Schreiner MM, Juras V, et al. Prediction of lumbar disk herniation and clinical outcome using quantitative magnetic resonance imaging: a 5-year follow-up study. Invest Radiol 2019;54(3):183–9.

15. Swärd L, Hellström M, Jacobsson B, et al. Disc degeneration and associated abnormalities of the spine in elite gymnasts. A magnetic resonance imaging study. Spine (Phila Pa 1976) 1991;16(4):437–43.

16. Abdalkader M, Guermazi A, Engebretsen L, et al. MRI-detected spinal disc degenerative changes in athletes participating in the Rio de Janeiro 2016 Summer Olympics games. BMC Musculoskelet Disord 2020;21(1):45.

17. Gray BL, Buchowski JM, Bumpass DB, et al. Disc herniations in the National Football League. Spine (Phila Pa 1976) 2013;38(22):1934–8.

18. Rajeswaran G, Turner M, Gissane C, et al. MRI findings in the lumbar spines of asymptomatic elite junior tennis players. Skeletal Radiol 2014;43(7):925–32.

19. Witwit WA, Kovac P, Sward A, et al. Disc degeneration on MRI is more prevalent in young elite skiers compared to controls. Knee Surg Sports Traumatol Arthrosc 2018;26(1):325–32.

20. Nachemson AL. Disc pressure measurements. Spine (Phila Pa 1976) 1981; 6(1):93–7.

21. Vroomen PC, de Krom MC, Wilmink JT, et al. Diagnostic value of history and physical examination in patients suspected of lumbosacral nerve root compression. J Neurol Neurosurg Psychiatr 2002;72(5):630–4.

22. Vucetic N, Svensson O. Physical signs in lumbar disc hernia. Clin Orthop Relat Res 1996;333:192–201.

23. Kreiner DS, Hwang SW, Easa JE, et al. An evidence-based clinical guideline for the diagnosis and treatment of lumbar disc herniation with radiculopathy. Spine J 2014;14(1):180–91.

24. Rabin A, Gerszten PC, Karausky P, et al. The sensitivity of the seated straight-leg raise test compared with the supine straight-leg raise test in patients presenting with magnetic resonance imaging evidence of lumbar nerve root compression. Arch Phys Med Rehabil 2007;88(7):840–3.

25. Janssen ME, Bertrand SL, Joe C, et al. Lumbar herniated disk disease: comparison of MRI, myelography, and post-myelographic CT scan with surgical findings. Orthopedics 1994;17(2):121–7.

26. Hsu WK, McCarthy KJ, Savage JW, et al. The Professional Athlete Spine Initiative: outcomes after lumbar disc herniation in 342 elite professional athletes. Spine J 2011;11(3):180–6.

27. Iwamoto J, Sato Y, Takeda T, et al. Return to play after conservative treatment in athletes with symptomatic lumbar disc herniation: a practice-based observational study. Open Access J Sports Med 2011;2:25–31.

28. Saal JA, Saal JS. Nonoperative treatment of herniated lumbar intervertebral disc with radiculopathy. An outcome study. Spine (Phila Pa 1976) 1989;14(4):431–7.
29. Weber H. The natural history of disc herniation and the influence of intervention. Spine (Phila Pa 1976) 1994;19(19):2234.
30. Watkins RG 3rd. Great rehabilitation and great physical bodies allow professional athletes undergoing lumbar discectomy to return to sport at a high rate. Spine J 2011;11(3):187–9.
31. Chou R, Deyo R, Friedly J, et al. Systemic pharmacologic therapies for low back pain: a systematic review for an American College of Physicians Clinical Practice Guideline. Ann Intern Med 2017;166(7):480–92.
32. Goldberg H, Firtch W, Tyburski M, et al. Oral steroids for acute radiculopathy due to a herniated lumbar disk: a randomized clinical trial. JAMA 2015;313(19): 1915–23.
33. Calandre EP, Rico-Villademoros F, Slim M. Alpha$_2$delta ligands, gabapentin, pregabalin and mirogabalin: a review of their clinical pharmacology and therapeutic use [published correction appears in Expert Rev Neurother. 2016 Nov;16(11):iii]. Expert Rev Neurother 2016;16(11):1263–77.
34. Enke O, New HA, New CH, et al. Anticonvulsants in the treatment of low back pain and lumbar radicular pain: a systematic review and meta-analysis. CMAJ 2018;190(26):E786–93.
35. Witenko C, Moorman-Li R, Motycka C, et al. Considerations for the appropriate use of skeletal muscle relaxants for the management of acute low back pain. P T 2014;39(6):427–35.
36. Ackerman WE 3rd, Ahmad M. The efficacy of lumbar epidural steroid injections in patients with lumbar disc herniations. Anesth Analg 2007;104(5):1217–22.
37. Taskaynatan MA, Tezel K, Yavuz F, et al. The effectiveness of transforaminal epidural steroid injection in patients with radicular low back pain due to lumbar disc herniation two years after treatment. J Back Musculoskeletal Rehabil 2015; 28(3):447–51.
38. Radcliff K, Hilibrand A, Lurie JD, et al. The impact of epidural steroid injections on the outcomes of patients treated for lumbar disc herniation: a subgroup analysis of the SPORT trial. J Bone Joint Surg Am 2012;94(15):1353–8.
39. Iwamoto J, Sato Y, Takeda T, et al. The return to sports activity after conservative or surgical treatment in athletes with lumbar disc herniation. Am J Phys Med Rehabil 2010;89(12):1030–5.
40. Weinstein JN, Tosteson TD, Lurie JD, et al. Surgical vs nonoperative treatment for lumbar disk herniation: the Spine Patient Outcomes Research Trial (SPORT): a randomized trial. JAMA 2006;296(20):2441–50.
41. Atlas SJ, Deyo RA, Keller RB, et al. The Maine Lumbar Spine Study, Part II. 1-year outcomes of surgical and nonsurgical management of sciatica. Spine (Phila Pa 1976) 1996;21(15):1777–86.
42. Clark AJ, Safaee MM, Khan NR, et al. Tubular microdiscectomy: techniques, complication avoidance, and review of the literature. Neurosurg Focus 2017; 43(2):E7.
43. Arts MP, Peul WC, Brand R, et al. Cost-effectiveness of microendoscopic discectomy versus conventional open discectomy in the treatment of lumbar disc herniation: a prospective randomised controlled trial [ISRCTN51857546]. BMC Musculoskelet Disord 2006;7:42.
44. Matsunaga S, Sakou T, Taketomi E, et al. Comparison of operative results of lumbar disc herniation in manual laborers and athletes. Spine (Phila Pa 1976) 1993; 18(15):2222–6.

45. Dohrmann GJ, Mansour N. Long-term results of various operations for lumbar disc herniation: analysis of over 39,000 patients. Med Princ Pract 2015;24(3): 285–90.
46. Lurie JD, Tosteson TD, Tosteson AN, et al. Surgical versus nonoperative treatment for lumbar disc herniation: eight-year results for the spine patient outcomes research trial [published correction appears in Spine (Phila Pa 1976). 2015 Jan;40(1):E59]. Spine (Phila Pa 1976) 2014;39(1):3–16.
47. Watkins RG 4th, Williams LA, Watkins RG 3rd. Microscopic lumbar discectomy results for 60 cases in professional and Olympic athletes. Spine J 2003;3(2): 100–5.
48. Minhas SV, Kester BS, Hsu WK. Outcomes after lumbar disc herniation in the National Basketball Association. Sports Health 2016;8(1):43–9.
49. Weistroffer JK, Hsu WK. Return-to-play rates in National Football League linemen after treatment for lumbar disk herniation. Am J Sports Med 2011;39(3): 632–6.
50. Schroeder GD, McCarthy KJ, Micev AJ, et al. Performance-based outcomes after nonoperative treatment, discectomy, and/or fusion for a lumbar disc herniation in National Hockey League athletes. Am J Sports Med 2013;41(11):2604–8.

Cervical Disc Herniations, Radiculopathy, and Myelopathy

Robert G. Watkins IV, MD*, Robert G. Watkins III, MD

KEYWORDS

- Cervical • Disc • Herniation • Radiculopathy • Myelopathy

KEY POINTS

- A burner in 1 arm probably is a nerve root injury and has a good prognosis. A burner in both arms probably is a spinal cord injury and requires significant work-up.
- Determining risk of return to play after transient paraparesis depends on severity of episode, number of episodes, and underlying anatomy.
- Fusion is the most common surgery performed in athletes because it has the safest chance to protect an injured nerve and allow for return to head contact in sports.
- Artificial disc replacement preserves motion and, therefore, may decrease the incidence of adjacent-level pathology but carries an unknown risk with head contact in sports.
- Posterior foraminotomy has the fastest healing and return to sports but the highest incidence of recurrent surgery at the index level.

INTRODUCTION

Treating high-level athletes requires the physician to deal with many confounding socioeconomic issues. A physician's abilities to take a history, perform a comprehensive physical examination, obtain diagnostic studies, direct the rehabilitation program, and receive proper follow-up often are compromised by many factors. The key to successful treatment depends on the physician's ability to overcome these obstacles and deliver the best possible care to each individual patient. The physician must be diligent and meticulous in order to make an accurate diagnosis, direct proper medical care, and follow-up with athletes on an ongoing basis. This article aims to help the medical team in providing comprehensive care for the elite athlete with spinal injury.

TRAUMATIC INJURIES
In-game Management

In preparation for treating athletes with acute injuries, the medical staff needs to have a plan that includes prevention strategies to reduce the incidence of cervical spine

Marina Spine Center, 4640 Admiralty Way, Suite 600, Marina del Rey, CA, 90292, USA
* Corresponding author.
E-mail address: robertwatkinsmd@yahoo.com

Clin Sports Med 40 (2021) 513–539
https://doi.org/10.1016/j.csm.2021.03.006
0278-5919/21/© 2021 Elsevier Inc. All rights reserved.

injuries in sport; emergency planning and preparation to increase management efficiency; maintaining or creating neutral alignment in the cervical spine; accessing and maintaining the airway; stabilizing and transferring the athlete with a suspected cervical spine injury; managing the athlete participating in equipment-laden sports, such as football, hockey, and lacrosse; understanding emergent transportation by whom and to where; and considerations in the emergency department.[1]

In American football, if a player is suspected of having a cervical spine injury on the field, it is important to engage in spinal precautions and leave the headgear in place until the cervical spine can be evaluated completely. The team personnel should have means available for removal of the face mask so that the airway is readily accessible. Immediate removal of the helmet should not be performed until the proper medical personnel are prepared for an emergency situation. When lifting a player with a suspected cervical injury, the physician should stabilize the head and neck to the torso by placing their hands under the scapulas and stabilizing the head between their forearms.

The team physician should have a high index of suspicion for a cervical spine injury for any player who goes down after a collision. If the player is unconscious, assume a cervical fracture. If the player has a stiff and painful neck, assume a cervical fracture. If the player has loss of sensation or motor in extremities, assume a cervical fracture. If any of these conditions is met, the player should be carted off the field on a spine board with cervical precautions.

If a player runs off the field on their own accord, but the sideline evaluation reveals limited range of motion, cervical tenderness, cervical radiculopathy with pain/weakness/numbness, or pain with head compression, then the player should be evaluated for possible fracture or disc herniation.

Burners/Stingers

The most common athletic cervical neurologic injuries are stingers, or burners. Symptoms result from injury to the brachial plexus or cervical nerve roots. Stingers have been reported to occur in up to 50% of athletes involved in contact or collision sports.[2] A stinger or burner (burner syndrome) is a nerve injury associated with burning arm pain and paresthesias. A stinger may start with severe pain in the neck and arm and then quickly proceeds to unilateral dysesthetic pain that follows a dermatomal distribution. It may be accompanied by weakness, most often in the muscle groups supplied by the C5 and C6 nerve roots (shoulder abduction, elbow flexion, wrist extension, and grip) on the affected side. Although pain frequently resolves spontaneously in 10 minutes to 15 minutes, it is not uncommon to have trace abnormal neurologic findings for several months. Normal, painless motion of the cervical spine generally is present and is crucial in distinguishing a stinger from other types of cervical pathology, such as disc herniation, foraminal stenosis, or fracture. Bilateral symptoms (burning into both hands) are more indicative of a neurapraxic injury of the spinal cord, which requires much more caution and work-up.

Three different mechanisms of a burner syndrome have been described:

1. The most common is hyperextension, rotation, and compression toward the involved arm, thereby closing the neural foramen and causing a nerve root contusion (**Fig. 1**). This mechanism essentially is a replication of Spurling maneuver.
2. Lateral neck flexion away from a shoulder depression injury, resulting in brachial plexus stretch, is more common in younger adolescents.
3. A direct blow to the brachial plexus with resultant injury.

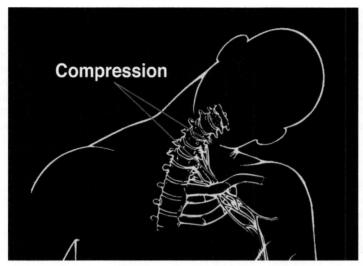

Fig. 1. Mechanism of stinger with ipsilateral cervical extension, rotation, and compression.

Most stingers resolve within minutes. For an athlete's first episode with only brief transitory symptoms, treatment is conservative and no special testing is required. The athlete is permitted to return to unrestricted activity after complete resolution of symptoms, if a normal neurologic examination, negative head compression test, and pain-free and unrestricted cervical range of motion are present. Further work-up is directed at patients with persistent symptoms or recurrent episodes to assess for other cervical problems, such as fracture, stenosis, disc herniation, or instability. Work-up includes cervical radiographs with supervised flexion-extension views, single-photon emission computed tomography (SPECT) bone scan (which can identify acute injury vs congenital anomaly), magnetic resonance imaging (MRI), computed tomography (CT) scan, and electromyography (EMG).

If the symptoms have not resolved by 3 weeks, it is reasonable to obtain an EMG. This test can help define the specific nerve root involved and determine the degree of injury. Because results of this test may lag behind an athlete's recovery, under certain circumstances, the player may be cleared to play when they are asymptomatic, even if the EMG has not returned normal.

Risk Categories by Sport

Sports can be categorized into several groups based on risk of injury: collision, contact, and repetitive.[3] Collision sports have the highest frequency and risk of head contact; examples include football, ice hockey, rugby, martial arts, and wrestling. These sports have the highest risk for cervical spine problems. A sport, such as football, that has a premium on yardage gained, has an inherent risk of lowering the head and using the crown of the head to initiate blows; therefore, it has an inherent risk for creating cervical fracture dislocations. Lowering of the head causes straightening of the spine and axial load being borne directly down the anterior spinal column, much like pushing the ends of a soda straw and having it buckle in the middle.[4]

Additional rules in football that attempt to eliminate use of the head as an offensive weapon were initiated to protect the person being hit, although in reality they protect the hitter from neck injury. Cervical injury is different in different sports, because a hockey player can be driven head first into the boards whereas in rugby there can be an unusual collapse of the scrum. Additionally, any sport in which a player can be dropped directly on their head has a significant risk of neck injury.

Contact sports are considered a medium risk for cervical injury.[3] Sports not designed for high velocity head contact, such as soccer, basketball, volleyball, baseball, and water polo, still can have a cervical injury but at a lower frequency. There also are high-velocity injuries in certain noncontact sports, such as skiing, gymnastics, and cheerleading. Repetitive sports that require a lot of cervical motion, such as golf, baseball, and swimming, can produce wear and tear injury to the cervical spine but with a lower risk of a catastrophic head contact injury.

Risk Categories by Condition

There are no universally accepted guidelines for determining when an athlete may return to play after a cervical injury. The ideal criteria include

- The athlete should be symptom-free with respect to neck and radicular pain.
- Unrestricted and pain-free cervical motion should be present.
- Neurologic evaluation should be normal.
- Full muscle strength should be present.
- There should be no evidence of radiographic instability or other spinal abnormalities on advanced imaging studies.

Often, patients have residual symptoms, physical findings, and/or anatomic conditions that increase risk for future injuries with return to athletic competition. Risk assessment can be helpful by dividing patients into the following categories, although each case needs to be assessed individually[5]:

Box 1
No contraindication to return to play

1. Posttraumatic
   - Healed, nondisplaced, stable C1 or C2 fracture (treated nonoperatively) with normal cervical range of motion.
   - Healed stable subaxial spine fracture with no sagittal plane kyphotic deformity
   - Asymptomatic clay shoveler fracture (C7 spinous process)

2. Congenital
   - Single-level Klippel-Feil syndrome (excluding the occipital–C1 articulation) with no evidence of instability or stenosis noted on MRI
   - Spinal bifida occulta

3. Degenerative
   - History of cervical degenerative disc disease that has been treated successfully in the clinical setting of occasional cervical neck stiffness with no change in baseline strength profile

4. Postsurgical
   - After anterior single-level cervical fusion (below C3-4), with or without instrumentation, that has healed
   - After single-level or multiple-level posterior cervical microlaminoforaminotomy

5. Other
   - Prior history of 2 stingers within the same or multiple seasons. The stingers should last less than 24 hours, and the athlete should have full range of cervical motion without any evidence of neurologic deficit.

---

1. No contraindications to return to play (**Box 1**): these conditions are considered to permit return to collision sports without restriction after comprehensive patient assessment.
2. Relative contraindications to return to play (**Box 2**): these conditions are associated with a possibility for recurrent injury despite the absence of any absolute contraindication. The athlete, family, and coach must be counseled that recurrent injury is a possibility and that the degree of risk is determined by each individual case.
3. Absolute contraindications to return to play (**Box 3**): these conditions most likely would not be allowed to return to collision sports.

OFFICE EVALUATION OF CERVICAL INJURIES

Athletes present to the clinic with cervical complaints that include neck pain, restricted range of motion, arm pain/weakness/numbness, balance disturbance, loss of fine motor control, and altered sensation in upper extremities affecting athletic performance. A detailed history and physical examination are essential to determine nerve root involvement (**Table 1**) and presence of myelopathy and to rule out other conditions. The physician must be able to make an accurate diagnosis, determine acuity and risk for injury, and provide a structured timeline for diagnostic studies, treatment, and return to play.

Head contact sports are at greatest risk for a cervical spine injury. Certain positions in certain sports involve repetitive axial loading of the cervical spine, which may cause acute injury and/or chronic degenerative changes. For example, in rugby, the front-line players in the scrum who sustain the largest loads and have higher rates of acute cervical spine injuries also had the highest incidence of severe cervical degenerative changes.[6] Additionally, in a sample of National Football League (NFL) retirees aged 30 years to 49 years, 37% self-reported a diagnosis of arthritis and pain in the neck compared with 17% in the general population.[7]

Box 2
Relative contraindication to return to play

1. Previous history of transient quadriplegia or quadriparesthesia. The athlete must have full return to baseline strength and cervical range of motion with no increase in baseline cervical neck discomfort and imaging evidence of no significant spinal cord compression.

2. Continued cervical neck discomfort or any evidence of a neurologic deficit or decreased range of motion from baseline after a cervical spine injury.

3. Three or more stingers in the same season

4. A prolonged stinger lasting more than 24 hours

5. A healed, displaced cervical fracture

6. A healed single-level posterior fusion with lateral mass segmental fixation

7. A healed single-level anterior fusion at C2-3 or C3-4 (sports that require head contact increase the risk of future injury, especially in a kyphotic spine)

8. A healed, stable, 2-level anterior or posterior cervical fusion with or without instrumentation (below C3-4) (sports that require head contact increase the risk of future injury)

9. A healed cervical laminoplasty (sports that require head contact increase the risk of future injury)

Box 3
Absolute contraindication to return to play

1. Previous transient quadriparesis
   - More than 2 previous episodes of transient quadriplegia or quadriparesthesia
   - Clinical history or physical findings of cervical myelopathy

2. Postsurgical
   - C1-2 cervical fusion
   - Three-level cervical spine fusion
   - Multilevel cervical laminectomy

3. Soft tissue injury or deficiencies
   - Asymptomatic ligamentous laxity (ie, >11° of kyphotic deformity compared with the cephalad or caudal vertebral level)
   - Radiographic evidence of C1-2 hypermobility with an anterior dens interval of 4 mm or greater
   - Radiographic evidence of a distraction-extension cervical spine injury
   - Symptomatic acute cervical disc herniation

4. Other radiographic findings
   - Plain radiography
     i. Evidence of a spear tackler spine on radiographic analysis and history
     ii. A multiple-level Klippel-Feil syndrome
     iii. Clinical or radiographic evidence of rheumatoid arthritis
     iv. Radiographic evidence of ankylosing spondylitis or diffuse idiopathic skeletal hyperostosis
     v. A healed subaxial spine fracture with evidence of a kyphotic sagittal plane or coronal plane abnormality
   - MRI
     i. Presence of cervical spinal cord abnormality noted on MRI.
     ii. MRI evidence of basilar invagination
     iii. MRI evidence of Arnold-Chiari malformation
     iv. MRI evidence of significant residual cord compression after a healed stable subaxial spine fracture
   - CT
     i. C1-2 rotatory fixation
     ii. Occipital–C1 assimilation

History

Patients with radiculopathy typically present with unilateral neck pain and radiation into the arm in a dermatomal distribution. The absence of pain in the arm, however, does not exclude the presence of radiculopathy. The most common symptom in cervical radiculopathy is radicular pain, followed by paresthesia. Weakness is reported by approximately 15% of patients.[8] In most cases, the affected nerve root can be identified by history and physical examination alone.[9] Patients often report worsening of symptoms with neck extension or rotation/lateral bending to the ipsilateral side. Pain referred to the medial border of the scapula usually is referred cervical pain but not necessarily radicular pain.[10] Red flags in the history include pain at night (tumor), weight loss (malignancy), fever (infection), urinary urgency (myelopathy), and global weakness/tremors/spasticity (neurologic disorder).

Physical Examination

Physical examination should test for neck range of motion, motor and sensory of extremities, reflexes, gait, and special maneuvers, including Spurling maneuver, shoulder abduction test, shoulder impingement, Adson, Phalen, and Tinel at wrist and

Table 1
Cervical radiculopathy

Nerve Root	Pain Distribution	Motor	Sensory	Reflex
C1, C2, C3	Side of face, neck	—	Side of face	—
C4	Lower neck	—	Cape distribution	—
C5	Lateral arm	Deltoid, biceps	Lateral arm	Biceps
C6	Lateral forearm, thumb	Biceps, wrist extension	Lateral forearm, thumb	Brachioradialis
C7	Dorsolateral forearm, middle finger	Triceps, thumb extension	Dorsal forearm, middle finger	Triceps
C8	Medial forearm, ulnar digits	Finger flexors, index finger extension	Medial forearm, ulnar digits	—
T1	Medial forearm	Finger intrinsics	Medial forearm	—

elbow. The most common physical examination findings in persons with cervical radiculopathy are painful neck movements and muscle spasm. Diminished deep tendon reflex is the most common objective neurologic finding, with triceps involvement being the most prevalent. Weakness is the next most common finding.[8] The most common nerve root affected is C7, followed by C6.[8,11,12] Yoss and colleagues[13] found that diminished reflexes were correlated most commonly to the pathology identified at surgery (82%), followed by motor weakness (77%), and diminished sensation (65%).

The Spurling maneuver involves passively moving the patient's neck into ipsilateral rotation and then extension and then applying gentle downward axial compression. If radicular pain is elicited at any point in maneuver, then it is stopped, and the other parts are not completed. The purpose of this test is to constrict the neural foramen; a positive result is the reproduction of radicular symptoms. A systematic review of physical examination maneuvers in the setting of cervical radiculopathy found that the Spurling maneuver was most sensitive and specific when rotation and extension were combined.[14]

The shoulder abduction test is similar in specificity to the Spurling maneuver, based on electrodiagnostic correlation.[12] The test involves placing the palm of the affected limb on top of or near a patient's head. A positive result is the relief of radicular symptoms. The shoulder abduction test checks for the relief of symptoms with shoulder abduction as the nerve is taken off tension. Often, there is a history of sleeping with the arm in the abducted position for pain relief.

Shoulder abduction relieves radicular symptoms but provokes shoulder arthropathy. Shoulder pathology must be considered and ruled out in these patients because shoulder girdle pain frequently is the most common presenting symptom of cervical radiculopathy.[15] Also, selective injections can be helpful in establishing a diagnosis.

When diagnosing a patient with radiculopathy, it is important to test for cervical myelopathy. Patients with myelopathy present with upper motor neuron signs, including hyperreflexia and changes in gait, and also have difficulty with fine motor tasks (handwriting, buttoning shirts, and so forth). Upper extremity myelopathy results from spinal cord compression at C4 and cephalad. It presents with loss of dexterity of fine motor movements of hands and physical examination shows hyperreflexia of upper extremities and positive Hoffman test (involuntary flexion movement of thumb and/or index finger with flicking of the middle finger down). Compression of the spinal cord caudal to C4 does not cause upper extremity myelopathy but may result in lower extremity myelopathy. This results in imbalance with heel to toe tandem gait, lower extremity hyperreflexia, clonus and positive Babinski sign.

Cervical radiculopathy must be distinguished from peripheral nerve entrapment or brachial plexopathy (**Table 2**). Patients also may present with peripheral entrapment and cervical radiculopathy, a phenomenon known as double crush. Physical findings to test for other peripheral nerve issues include infraspinatus atrophy from suprascapular nerve compression, scapular winging from long thoracic nerve pathology, and deltoid weakness from axillary nerve injury. Other items on the differential diagnosis include cardiac pain, herpes zoster (shingles), infection, neurologic disorders (Guillain-Barré and amyotrophic lateral sclerosis) and intraspinal and extraspinal tumors.[16]

Diagnostic Evaluation

Initial diagnostic studies, such as radiographs and MRI, are performed when an athlete has a neurologic deficit, has radicular pain, or is not responding to conservative management. If a disc herniation is present on MRI, the physician needs to determine its acuity. The prevalence of cervical disc herniation in the asymptomatic population may be up to 25% for those younger than 40 years.[17] If a player has acute symptoms that

Table 2
Conditions that mimic cervical radiculopathy

Condition	Clinical Examination	Diagnostic Evaluation
Anterior interosseus nerve entrapment	Grip and pinch weakness, no pain	EMG
Arteriovenous malformation	Numbness, paresthesias, variable pain, weakness	MRI, ultrasound
Carpal tunnel syndrome	Numbness in radial 3.5 fingers, paresthesias, thenar weakness	1. No triceps, wrist extensor, or thumb extensor weakness 2. Tinel sign and Phalen test 3. EMG
Cubital tunnel syndrome	Flexor digitorum profundus weakness, numbness in ulnar half of ring and little fingers, paresthesias	1. No thumb interphalangeal weakness 2. Tinel sign test 3. EMG
Parsonage-Turner syndrome (brachial plexopathy)	Pain; then numbness and/or weakness in multiple nerve roots	EMG
Posterior interosseus nerve entrapment	Pain; wrist and finger extensor weakness	No triceps or wrist flexor weakness
Radial tunnel syndrome	Pain only in forearm	Diagnostic injection
Thoracic outlet syndrome	Pain, swelling, vascular insufficiency	1. Adson test 2. Angiography

correlate with the herniation on MRI and the morphology of the herniation appears acute (irregular or light on T2 image), then treatment and restriction on return to play are more conservative to help prevent worsening of the herniation.

There are 3 main types of cervical disc herniation. The most common is intraforaminal, which results in predominantly sensory radicular symptoms. The next most common is posterolateral, which results in weakness and potentially muscle atrophy. Rarer midline herniations directly compress the spinal cord and result in symptoms of myelopathy. Acute midline herniations need to be treated more cautiously in head contact sports because exacerbation of the herniation may cause spinal cord injury. In NFL players, Gray and colleagues[18] showed C3-4 and C5-6 to have the highest incidence of disc herniations, followed by C4-5.

Oblique MRI cuts are helpful to visualize nerve impingement in the foramen. Additionally, MRI may reveal cervical stenosis and pathology in the spinal cord. Spinal cord signal changes include high-signal intensity on T2, indicative of edema and better prognosis, and low-signal intensity on T1, indicative of necrosis and worse prognosis.

In cases of MRI that cannot be performed or are equivocal in determining nerve root impingement, a CT myelogram may be utilized. Furthermore, CT scans are better suited to the evaluation of bony pathology, may be used to better delineate hard disc impingement, and may contribute to type of surgery decision.[19,20]

Additionally, if radiographs and MRI do not explain the symptoms, a bone scan with cervical SPECT and CT merge can be obtained to demonstrate a stress fracture. The CT-SPECT merge also is helpful for differentiating between acute injuries and congenital anomalies, especially in the occiput to C2 region.

EMG and nerve conduction studies, performed after 3 weeks of neurologic deficit, can be helpful along with a detailed motor examination to distinguish radiculopathy from peripheral nerve injury. EMG used without imaging, however, has been shown to be a relatively poor tool for localization with only 42% of EMG findings correlated to findings at the time of surgery.[21]

Treatment

Cervical disc herniations in athletes is a common occurrence. Often the episode starts with pain and/or stiffness without any arm or radicular symptoms. Activities that provoke pain should be avoided in the first 1 week to 2 weeks of acute neck pain, to prevent an annular tear from becoming a herniation.

For moderate pain, nonsteroidal anti-inflammatory drugs are the first line of treatment. They have both analgesic and anti-inflammatory effects.[22] Oral anti-inflammatories are relatively benign and typically do not mask a significant annular tear in the disc.

For more severe pain, oral corticosteroids are used in the acute phase to manage the inflammatory cascade. Oral prednisone may mask inflammatory pain, and the medical staff should be more cautious about returning a player to the sport while still requiring prednisone in the acute phase of an injury. Degree of injury, physical findings, radiographic findings, response to treatment, completion of rehabilitation program, and response to gradual return to athletic activities are factors that determine time to return to play.

Cervical epidurals are used for significant pain that is not responding to oral medications. In the general population, good-quality evidence supports steroid injections for cervical radiculopathy caused by disc herniation but only fair evidence for radiculopathy caused by spondylosis.[23] In the authors' practice cervical epidurals are used for pain but not to treat a painless weakness. Typically, an athlete should not return to their sport for at least several days following an epidural for an acute problem.

Traction and manipulation commonly are used in athletic training rooms as part of treatment of cervical pathology. Neither one has significant data to support their use; however, both can be performed safely and effectively.[24–26] Care must be taken with both to not cause pathology, such as vertebral artery dissection, and, in the presence of acute herniation or myelopathy, to not worsen the condition.[15]

Predicting the time for return to play with an acute cervical radiculopathy is challenging. Sometimes, symptoms are mild, MRI findings appear stable, and the player returns to normal function in several days. Other times, the disc herniation may take 6 weeks to heal, the neurologic recovery may take 6 weeks to 12 weeks, the symptoms may persist for 6 weeks to 12 weeks, and the return to sport may take 3 months to 6 months.

With acute disc herniations, the general time estimate for return to play is 6 weeks. Factors considered detrimental to early return to play include: neurologic deficit (weakness), severe pain, and MRI findings, such as large herniation (5 mm), significant nerve compression, underlying stenosis, and spinal cord signal change (high-signal change on T2 or low-signal change on T1).

Rehabilitation is initiated once the pain is tolerable. Trunk stabilization and chest-out posture exercises can be performed without increasing intradiscal pressure. These exercises reinforce ideal posture, which brings the head back over the body, thereby increasing intervertebral foraminal height and decreasing the force of the head on the spine. The rehabilitation program starts with lumbar trunk stabilization exercises, thereby establishing a neutral pain-free core, and then proceeds to scapula stabilization and chest-out posture exercises. A well-designed physical therapy program should progress the patients through these stages as pain improves, beginning with gentle range of motion, core stabilization, and chest-out posturing, adding strengthening and conditioning activities once the acute symptoms subside.[15]

The comprehensive rehabilitation program is available in The Back Doctor app.[27] The player should obtain level 2 of the Back Program (**Fig. 2**) before initiating level 1 of the Neck Program and shoulder exercises. The player should obtain level 3 of the Back Program before initiating level 2 of the Neck Program and performing sport-specific exercises and activities, such as running, shooting, skating, throwing, hitting, and weight-lifting. The player should complete level 4 of the Back Program and level 2 of the Neck Program before returning to practice with the team. Return to sport requires completion of level 4 to level 5 of the Back Program, completion of level 2 of the Neck Program, completion of sport-specific exercises, adequate aerobic conditioning, gradual increase in minutes, and continuation of the rehabilitation program after returning to sport. The best reinjury prevention is to be in peak condition and performance.

SURGERY
Cervical Stenosis Surgery

Underlying cervical stenosis increases the chance of having symptoms and potentially undergoing surgery after an acute disc herniation. Stenosis typically is determined by MRI or CT myelogram. Functional spinal stenosis, defined as the loss of cerebrospinal fluid around the cord or deformation of the spinal cord, generally is more accurate and relevant than bony stenosis.[28] In the general population, cervical stenosis has been shown to increase the risk for permanent spinal cord injury after a fracture dislocation injury.[29,30] In football players, cervical stenosis has been shown to increase the risk for recurrent episodes of cord neuropraxia.[31] Episodes of neuropraxia, however, as an independent factor, have not been shown to increase the risk of permanent spinal cord

	Level 1	Level 2	Level 3	Level 4	Level 5
Dead Bug	Supported Arms, Marching Legs, 2 Min. or Supported Legs, Extended Arms, 2 Min.	Unsupported, Alternate Opposite Arms & Legs, 3 Min.	Unsupported, Alternate Opposite Arms & Legs, 7 Min.	Unsupported, Alternate Opposite Arms & Legs, 10 Min. May Add Weights.	Unsupported, Alternate Opposite Arms & Legs, 15 Min. May Add Weights.
Partial Sit-Up	Forward, Hands on Chest, 10 Reps.	Forward, Hands on Chest, 3 Sets x 10 Reps.	Hands Behind Head; Forward, Right, Left: 3 Sets x 10 Reps.	Weight on Chest: Forward, Right, Left: 3 Sets x 20 Reps.	Weights Overhead: Forward, Right, Left: 3 Sets x 30 Reps.
Bridging	Double Leg Supported, 2 Sets x 10 Reps.	Double Leg Supported 2 Sets x 20 Reps. May Add Weights to Hips	Single Leg Supported, Alternate Opposite Leg Extended, 3 Sets x 20 Reps, Each Side.	On Ball, Single Leg Extended, 4 Sets x 20 Reps, Each Side.	On Ball, Single Leg Extended, 5 Sets x 20 Reps, Each Side. With Ankle Weights.
Prone	Alternating Arm or Leg Lifts, 1 Set x 10 Reps. Hold 2 Sec.	Alternating Opposite Arm and Leg Lifts, 2 Sets x 10 Reps, Hold 5 Sec. Each Side.	On Ball: Flys, Swim, Supermans: 2 Sets x 20 Reps, Hold 5 Sec.	On Ball: Flys, Swim, Supermans w/ Weights, 2 Sets x 20 Reps. Walkout/pushups 3 Sets x 5 Reps.	On Ball: Flys, Swim, Supermans w/ Weights, 4 Sets x 20 Reps. Walkout/pushups 4 Sets x 10 Reps.
Quadruped	Alternate Arm or Leg, 1 Set x 10 Reps, Hold 2 Sec. Each Side.	Alternating Opposite Arm and Leg, 2 Sets x 10 Reps, Hold 5 Sec. Each Side.	Alternating Opposite Arm and Leg, 2 Sets x 20 Reps, Hold 5 Sec, Each Side.	Alternating Opposite Arm and Leg, 3 Sets x 20 Reps, Hold 5 Sec., w/ Weights.	Alternating Opposite Arm and Leg, 3 Sets x 20 Reps, Hold 15 Sec., w/ Weights.
Wall Slide	45 Degrees, 10 Reps, Hold 5 Sec.	90 Degrees, 10 Reps x 20 Sec.	90 Degrees, 10 Reps x 30 Sec. Lunges 1 Min.	90 Degrees, Weights at Side, 10 Reps x 30 Sec. Lunges w/ Weights at Side 3 Min.	90 Degrees, Weights with Arms Extended, 10 Reps x 30 Sec. Lunges w/ Weights in Front 5 Min.

Fig. 2. Categorization of levels in Back Program in Back Doctor app.

injury.[32] Typically, asymptomatic cervical stenosis is not treated prophylactically with surgery.

Return to play after an episode of transient neuropraxia depends on the degree of stenosis, presence of spinal cord compression or cord signal abnormalities, severity of acute injury (ie, quadriparesis lasting >36 h), signs and symptoms on examination, and risk for future injury. The physician's jobs are counseling the athlete on potential risks and making a recommendation of treatment. Cervical fusions may be performed if the degree of stenosis, degree of symptoms, biomechanics of the spine, and patient demographics determine that the risk of future injury is less post-fusion than with nonoperative management.

Fusion is the most common surgery performed on athletes for cervical spinal cord compression because it decompresses the disc herniation, restores room available for the cord with distraction, stops motion and spinal cord irritability, and prevents future injury at the index level. In the general population, artificial disc replacement (ADR) has shown promising results in relieving myelopathy due to anterior pathology.[33,34] Similarly, cervical laminoplasty is a motion-preserving operation that is appropriate for multilevel stenosis. In high-level sports, the risk of head contact after ADR and laminoplasty is unknown.

After cervical surgery, a player's ability to return to sport depends on resolution of symptoms, radiologic evidence of successful surgery, risk of future injury, and completion of the spinal rehabilitation program. At times, the player may have a successful surgery but may not return to sport because of multiple injuries at the end of their career or the desire to not risk future injury. Additionally, a player may be cleared to return to sport but may not get hired by a team.

Cervical Radiculopathy Surgery

Surgery is reserved for disc herniations and/or foraminal stenosis that do not respond to conservative management. Factors that determine the need and urgency for surgery include neurologic deficit, degree of pain with and without sport, degree of pathology, functional deficit, timing of season, status of athletic career, and risks and outcomes of the surgery. Factors to consider regarding a neurologic deficit include degree that the deficit effects performance and career, degree that the deficit effects activities of daily living without the sport, and response of the deficit to time and nonoperative care. In general, if a neurologic deficit is improving on a weekly basis, then surgical intervention is less likely to be needed. If weakness is not improving, then the chance of neurologic recovery is better if the surgery is done sooner rather than later. Studies have shown that a longer duration of symptoms preoperatively corresponds to worse outcomes after surgery.[35,36]

Surgical intervention for disc herniations and/or foraminal stenosis includes fusion (anterior cervical discectomy and fusion [ACDF]), ADR, and posterior foraminotomy (PF)/discectomy. Fusions are the most common surgery performed for cervical pathology, because the surgery directly decompresses the nerve with minimal neurologic manipulation, distracts the foramen, stops the motion of the segment, and prevents recurrence of symptoms from the fused level. The downsides of cervical fusions include time to bony healing, risk of nonunion, and risk of pathology at adjacent levels that may result in long-term neck pain or adjacent-level nerve compression. Incidence of adjacent-level disease after fusion in athletes has been reported to be 5% to 10%.[37,38]

Fusion Results

In the general population, recent data on ACDF in cervical radiculopathy have been obtained from studies of cervical disc arthroplasty.[39–43] These were multicenter prospective randomized trials with follow-up ranging from 4 years to 6 years. After fusion, these studies show a significant and durable improvement in clinical outcomes with neurologic success of 89%.[43] Implant-related complications in the fusion groups were 7%. Additionally, in the fusion patients, there was a 12% rate of secondary procedures by the 4-years to 6-year follow-up interval, with a 10% reoperation rate at the index level and 9% rate of operation at the adjacent level.

In addition to adjacent-level pathology, pseudarthrosis remains a concern following ACDF. A recent meta-analysis reported an overall pseudarthrosis rate of 2.6%; 0.9% when autograft was used and 4.8% when allograft was used.[44] In athletes, the authors typically use a titanium-coated polyetheretherketone spacer filled with iliac crest cancellous autograft and a 4-screw plate.

Return to Play after Fusion

A review of the literature by Dailey concludes that "surgical fixation with single-level ACDF to eliminate single-level neurologic compression causing radiculopathy or myelopathy is a strong recommendation as a treatment option to return to full contact sports play."[45] This recommendation is based primarily on 1 cohort study of 17 players who underwent ACDF in which an increased incidence of catastrophic injury was not seen. Additional reports support a low risk of return to play after a single-level ACDF.[5,46–48] Specifically, McAnany and colleagues[49] showed that return to play following ACDF in professional contact athletes was 73.5%.

Watkins and colleagues[38] reported on 26 professional athletes who underwent 27 ACDF surgeries. By sport, categorization was 13, NFL; 5, National Hockey League;

5, Major League Baseball; 3, National Basketball Association; and 1, Major League Soccer: 26 of 27 (96.3%) showed clinical and radiographic evidence of fusion and 20 of 25 eligible players returned to play (80%). Average time to return to play in a professional game was 9.5 months. The incidence of adjacent-level pathology after a single-level fusion was 8%.

Maroon and colleagues[48] reported on 15 athletes, 7 NFL players and 8 wrestlers, after single-level ACDF, with a return to play of 87% at average 6 months (range 2–12 mo). Of the NFL players, 5 of 7 returned to play (71%). The 2 players who did not return to play were cleared from a spinal perspective but retired due to orthopedic injuries. One NFL player who returned to play subsequently retired after sustaining a disc herniation at an adjacent level.

In a study of 19 professional rugby players, Andrews and colleagues[46] showed 13 of 17 (76%) single-level ACDF players returned to play. Both players with 2-level ACDF had difficulties and did not return to play. Furthermore, 15% of the single-level ACDF players who returned to play experienced future symptoms.

In the authors' experience, many NFL players with herniations and/or stenosis at C3-4 have a loss of lordosis centered at this level. Under axial loading, the neck typically fails in flexion,[50,51] and a kyphotic segment increases the risk of a flexion injury. During a head-down tackle, the compressive impact may be up to 98 times the force of gravity delivered axially to the cervical spine.[28] A fusion of C3-4 at the middle of a straight or kyphotic segment in a head contact position may put significant stress on the C2-3 segment. The risk of catastrophic spinal cord injury at C2-3 and/or chronic pain from future occipital to C3 degeneration needs to be considered before returning a head contact athlete to play after a C3-4 fusion.

Maroon and colleagues[52] have reported on 3 NFL players who underwent fusion at C3-4 who had a T2 hyperintense lesion in the spinal cord preoperative. Two of 3 returned to play successfully; the third still was awaiting final clearance. The investigators concluded in this study that "MRI T2 hyper-intensity in contact sport athletes (treated surgically or non-operatively) who are symptom-free with normal examination and no evidence of spinal instability may not be a contraindication to return to play."

Multilevel Fusion

Data are lacking on the safety of return to sport after a 2-level neck fusion. There is a report of a professional rugby player and 2 military men who returned successfully after 2-level ACDF.[53] Conversely, Andrews and colleagues46 reported on 2 rugby players who struggled on return to play after a 2-level fusion. Additionally, there is a catastrophic case report of a rugby player 2 years after a 2-level ACDF at C5-6 and C6-7, in which the player suffered a C3-4 facet dislocation and complete impairment with C5 cord injury.[54] This demonstrates the significant risk and return after multilevel fusion to a collision or contact sport.

In professional sports in which head contact is probable and inherent in the sport, such as football and other collision sports, return to play after 2-level ACDF generally is not recommended. In a non–head contact sport (eg, baseball or basketball), a player may be cleared to return to sport after a 2-level neck fusion. At times, however, the authors have not recommended a 2-level neck fusion in player in order to return to sport. In other words, if they are relatively asymptomatic with life outside of sports, sometimes the authors do not recommend a 2-level neck fusion in order to have a chance to return to sports. Although there are some data on adjacent-level pathology after multilevel neck fusion for degenerative disc disease, there are no data on 20-year-old to 30-year-old people after traumatic disc herniations undergoing multilevel fusions. The authors' concern is the risk for long-term lack of mobility, adjacent-level pathology, and chronic pain.

Posterior Foraminotomy

PF avoids the complications of fusions but has a higher chance of residual or recurrent symptoms from the surgical level. Mai and colleagues[37] reported on 101 professional athletes undergoing cervical spine surgery (ACDF = 86, PF = 13, and total disc replacement = 2). The PF cohort had a significantly greater return to play rate and shortest time to return after surgery. The reoperation rate at the index level, however, was significantly higher in PF athletes compared with ACDF athletes (46.2% vs 5.8%, respectively; $P < .001$). The operation rate after ACDF for adjacent-level pathology was 4.7% (4/86).

In the general population, studies have shown the PF to be an effective surgery with durable long-term outcome.[55–58] One long-term study reported a reoperation rate of 10% at an average of 2.4 years' follow-up; however, reoperations reached 18% and 24%, respectively, when minimum 2-year and 10-year follow-ups were considered.[55] In this series, 91% of patients experienced symptom improvement at 1 month, and 85% had improvement at an average of 4-year follow-up. A multivariate analysis revealed that preoperative neck pain was an independent predictor of reoperation. Another study reported a lower rate of reoperation after PF (1.1% per index level per year and 0.9% per adjacent-level per year).[56]

PF is an alternative to fusion, especially in multilevel pathology, and has shown durable long-term results in the general population. The authors may choose to do a foraminotomy if the patient has significant multilevel disease where the risk for adjacent-level pathology is more significant after a fusion. In the authors' experience, the foraminotomy is most effective if the patient gets relief of radicular symptoms with shoulder abduction.

In patients referred to the authors, 1 recurrent disc herniation with radiculopathy after posterior discectomy and 2 cases of fracture after foraminotomy in professional football players have been seen. The fractures occurred in the lateral masses at the index level. Both fractures healed with conservative care. The players (linebacker and defensive back) did not return to professional competition. The important factor in foraminotomy probably is the method used for the foraminotomy. The more bone removed, the greater the risk of recurrent injury at that level.

The authors have used a minimally invasive decompressive technique, preserving the facet joint, detaching the ligament, and decompressing the undersurface of the joint as a minimal bone removal technique for burners and stingers in professional athletes.[59] The authors have not used PF and discectomy for disc herniations in professional athletes, which the authors believe require more facet removal. Additionally, on surgical patients, the authors have had players who sustain repetitive blows to the head (such as offensive linemen) who have had difficulty after PF.

Artificial Disc Replacement

Choosing between a fusion, ADR, and PF depends on many factors. In the authors' practice, if an athlete has a functional neurologic deficit and normal adjacent segments, a fusion has the best chance of treating the immediate pathology with low risk of additional problems. If an athlete has multilevel pathology and/or kyphosis, the risks after fusion increase; therefore, PF may be a more ideal treatment. The stability of an ADR in a head contact sport is undetermined at this point. There have been reports of failures after ADR.[60,61] An ADR may be acceptable in a contact sport, such as baseball, but the risk for violent collisions still exist and pose a risk for dislodgement.

A fusion is most reliable to treat an injured nerve at the index level because of the foraminal distraction, stoppage of motion, and preservation of neurologic decompression. Studies of the general population, however, have indicated similar, if not slightly better, neurologic recovery after artificial disc compared with fusion.[61–63] This may be because surgeons perform a more thorough direct decompression during an artificial disc surgery compared with the fusion surgery.

The literature summary of ADR compared with fusion in the general population: ADR is an alternative to fusion for cervical degenerative disc disease given outcomes that statistically are noninferior to fusion: perioperative outcomes, health-related quality of life, patient satisfaction, treatment of myelopathy, and overall treatment success for 1-level cervical degenerative disc disease. ADR might be preferable to fusion for cervical degenerative disc disease, given outcomes that are statistically superior to fusion: quicker recovery and return to work, higher technical success and lower rate of reoperation at the index site, maintenance of more normal spinal segment kinetics, and higher overall treatment success for 2-level cervical degenerative disc disease.[33,34,64,65]

Return to Play

Return to play after cervical spine surgery depends on healing of the surgical structures, neurologic recovery, and rehabilitation. A foraminotomy for posterior foraminal stenosis has the least significant anatomic structures to heal. The cervical muscles and facet capsule may heal in 4 weeks to 6 weeks. A posterior discectomy probably takes longer for the annular defect to heal, approximately 6 weeks to 10 weeks. An ADR takes approximately 12 weeks for bony ingrowth. A fusion typically takes 3 months to 6 months to heal. The time for the surgical structures to heal does not equal return to play. The athlete must complete a well-organized rehabilitation and sport-specific program prior to return.

When the postoperative pain has subsided (typically 4 weeks to 6 weeks), physical therapy and rehabilitation begin. The athlete must establish neutral spine stabilization before progressing to balance and coordination exercises. Sport-specific exercises gradually are introduced as long as the athlete remains asymptomatic. Return to sport after surgery follows the same protocol as described previously for nonoperative care. Return requires completion of rehabilitation program, sport-specific training, cardiovascular training, and gradual return to full competition.

Box 4
Collison sports: return to play after surgery

- ACDF: 1 level = probable RTP
- Foraminotomy: 1 level, 2 level, or 3 level = probable RTP
- ACDF: 2 level = not likely RTP
- ADR: 1 level = depends on risk for potential injury to index level
- Laminoplasty = not likely RTP

Abbreviation: RTP, return to play.

> **Box 5**
> **Contact sports: return to play after surgery**
>
> - Foraminotomy: 1 level, 2 level, or 3 level = most likely RTP
> - ACDF: 1 level = most likely RTP
> - ACDF: 2 level = probable RTP
> - Laminoplasty = possible RTP
> - ADR: 1 level = probable RTP
> - ADR 2 level = possible RTP

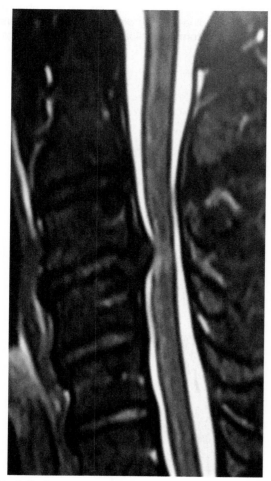

Fig. 3. Sagittal MRI of disc herniation at C3-4.

Performance After Surgery

There are limited data on performance after return for individual sports. Hsu[47] reported on NFL athletes undergoing operative and nonoperative treatment of cervical disc herniation. In the operative group, on average, 38 of 53 (72%) players successfully returned to play for 29 games over a 2.8-year period, which was significantly greater than that of the nonoperative group, in which only 21 of 46 (46%) players successfully returned to the field to play after treatment of 15 games over a 1.5-year period ($P = .04$). Performance scores and the percentage of games started were not statistically significantly different for either cohort, before and after treatment. Maroon and colleagues[66] found a similar average length of time played (3 years) after ACDF in NFL players. Roberts and colleagues[67] showed that pitchers with cervical disc herniation treated operatively (7 ACDF and 1 ADR) had no significant differences in performance-based outcomes postoperative compared with preoperative.

Risk of Return to Play

Risk stratification for return to play in collision sports are described previously. Likelihood of return to play after spine surgery depends on may factors, including age, sport, position, residual symptoms, physical examination findings, completion of

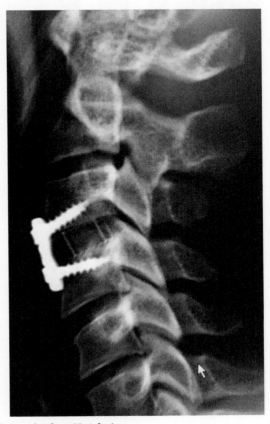

Fig. 4. Lateral radiograph after C3-4 fusion.

rehabilitation program, type of surgery, spinal level of surgery, current anatomy (kyphosis, rotation, stenosis, myelomalacia, stability, fusion, and adjacent-level pathology), and psychologic and social issues. The risks of future injury and long-term sequelae need to be discussed and determined by the surgeon and player on an individual case basis. **Boxes 4** and **5** provide an estimate for return to play after spine surgery for collision and contact sports.

CASES

Case 1 is an NFL linebacker who suffered transitory quadriparetic episode with herniation at C3-4 (**Fig. 3**). He underwent ACDF with resection of the herniation (**Fig. 4**). Although asymptomatic, the authors advised no return to play because of the high level of the injury and the cord contusion.

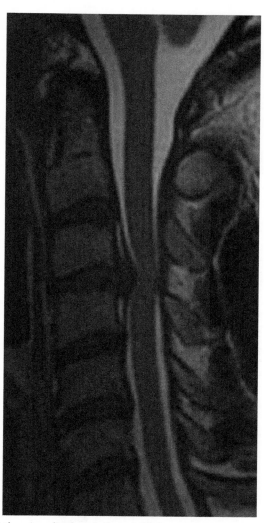

Fig. 5. Sagittal MRI showing disc herniation at C3-4.

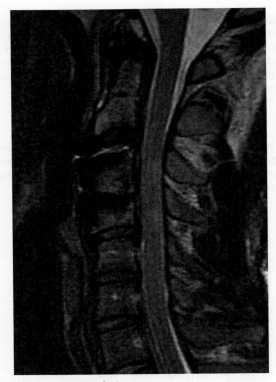

Fig. 6. Sagittal MRI 1-year post–C3-4 fusion.

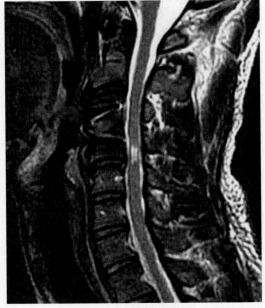

Fig. 7. Sagittal MRI 5 years post–C3-4 fusion, with myelomalacia at C4-5.

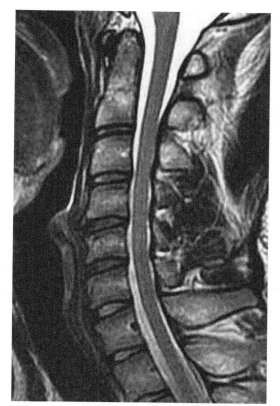

Fig. 8. Sagittal MRI of NCAA basketball player with transient paraparetic event.

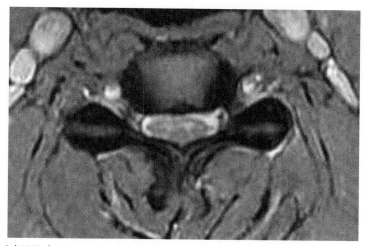

Fig. 9. Axial MRI showing congenital stenosis.

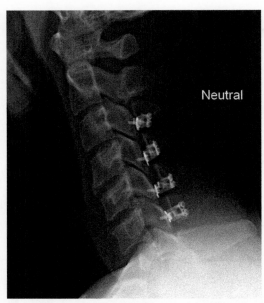

Fig. 10. Lateral radiograph after cervical laminoplasty.

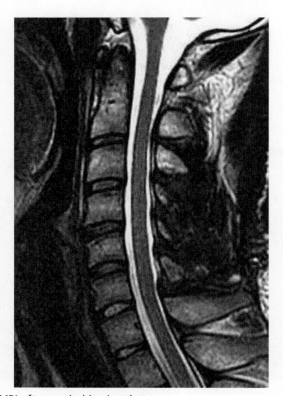

Fig. 11. Sagittal MRI after cervical laminoplasty.

Case 2 is an NBA guard who presented with a transitory quadriparetic episode (**Fig. 5**), treated with a C3-4 ACDF that resolved the spinal cord compression and kyphotic deformity (**Fig. 6**). Five years after surgery, while setting a pick in the NBA, contact incurred that produced a transitory quadriparetic episode secondary to a cord contusion at the level below the prior surgery (**Fig. 7**). The authors recommended retirement.

Case 3 is a National Collegiate Athletic Association (NCAA) basketball player with multiple episodes of transient quadriparesis whose cervical spine demonstrates congenital stenosis (**Figs. 8** and **9**). This patient underwent a 4-level cervical lamino-plasty (**Figs. 10** and **11**) and returned to play without the symptoms. In the determination of whether someone can return to play after cervical laminoplasty, the guidelines are ill defined at this time. It is contraindicated in a collision sport.

SYNOPSIS

The key to successful treatment of elite athletes is optimizing the medical care at every step: injury prevention and sport-specific training; comprehensive history and physical examination; high-quality and complete diagnostic studies; accurate diagnosis; control and completion of rehabilitation program; minimally invasive, safe, and effective surgeries; risk assessment for return to sport; guided and gradual return to sport; and continued rehabilitation and exercise program after return to sport.

CLINICS CARE POINTS

- A burner in 1 arm probably is a nerve root injury and has a good prognosis. A burner in both arms probably is a spinal cord injury and requires significant work-up.
- Determining risk of return to play after transient paraparesis depends on severity of episode, number of episodes, and underlying anatomy.
- Fusion is the most common surgery performed in athletes because it has the safest chance to protect an injured nerve and allow for return to head contact in sports.
- ADR preserves motion and, therefore, may decrease the incidence of adjacent-level pathology but carries an unknown risk with head contact in sports.
- PF has the fastest healing and return to sports but the highest incidence of recurrent surgery at the index level.

DISCLOSURE

The authors have nothing to disclose.

REFERENCES

1. Swartz EE, Boden BP, Courson RW, et al. National Athletic Trainers' Association position statement: acute management of the cervical spine–injured athlete. J Athl Train 2009;44(3):306–31.
2. Bowles RD, Canseco JA, Alexander TD, et al. The Prevalence and Management of Stingers in College and Professional Collision Athletes. Curr Rev Musculoskelet Med 2020. https://doi.org/10.1007/s12178-020-09665-5.
3. Morganti C, Sweeney CA, Albanese SA, et al. Return to play after cervical spine injury. Spine 2001;26:1131–6.

4. Schneider RC, Schemm GW. Vertebral artery insufficiency in acute and chronic spinal trauma, with special reference to the syndrome of acute central cervical spinal cord injury. J Neurosurg 1961;348–60.

5. Vaccaro AR, Watkins RG, Albert TJ, et al. Cervical spine injuries in athletes: return to play criteria. Orthopedics 2001;24:699–705.

6. Scher AT. Premature onset of degenerative disease of the cervical spine in rugby players. S Afr Med J 1990;77:557–8.

7. Weir Dr, Jackson JS, Sonnega A. University of Michigan Institute for social research, National Football League Player Care Foundation Study of Retired NFL Players. 2009. Available at: http://www.ns.umich.edu/Releases/2009/Sep09/FinalReport.pdf. Accessed May 17, 2020.

8. Radhakrishnan K, Litchy WJ, O'Fallon WM, et al. Epidemiology of cervical radicul-opathy. Brain 1994;117(pt 2):325–35.

9. Kuijper B, Tans JT, van der Kallen BF, et al. Root compression on MRI compared with clinical findings in patients with recent onset cervical radiculopathy. J Neurol Neurosurg Psychiatr 2011;82(5):561–3.

10. Levine MJ, Albert TJ, Smith MD. Cervical radiculopathy: diagnosis and nonoper-ative management. J Am Acad Orthop Surg 1996;4(6):305–16.

11. Ghasemi M, Golabchi K, Mousavi SA, et al. The value of provocative tests in diag-nosis of cervical radiculopathy. J Res Med Sci 2013;18(suppl 1):S35–8.

12. Vallée JN, Feydy A, Carlier RY, et al. Chronic cervical radiculopathy: lateral-approach periradicular corticosteroid injection. Radiology 2001;218(3):886–92.

13. Yoss RE, Corbin KB, MAcCarty CS, et al. Significance of symptoms and signs in localization of involved root in cervical disk protrusion. Neurology 1957;7:673–83.

14. Rubinstein SM, Pool JJ, vanTulder MW, et al. A systematic review of the diag-nostic accuracy of provocative tests of the neck for diagnosing cervical radicul-opathy. Eur Spine J 2007;16:307–19.

15. Rhee JM, Yoon T, Riew KD. Cervical radiculopathy. J Am Acad Orthop Surg 2007; 15:486–94.

16. Eubanks JD. Cervical radiculopathy: nonoperative management of neck pain and radicular symptoms. Am Fam Physician 2010;81:33–40.

17. Boden SD, McCowin PR, Davis DO, et al. Abnormal magnetic-resonance scans of the cervical spine in asymptomatic subjects. A prospective investigation. J Bone Joint Surg Am 1990;72:1178–84.

18. Gray BL, Buchowski JM, Bumpass DB, et al. Disc herniations in the National Foot-ball League. Spine 2013;38(22):1934–8.

19. Modic MT, Masaryk TJ, Ross JS, et al. Cervical radiculopathy: value of oblique MR imaging. Radiology 1987;163(1):227–31.

20. Bartlett RJ, Hill CR, Gardiner E. A comparison of T2 and gadolinium enhanced MRI with CT myelography in cervical radiculopathy. Br J Radiol 1998; 71(841):11–9.

21. Caridi JM, Pumberger M, Hughes AP. Cervical radiculopathy: a review. HSS J 2011;7:265–72.

22. Dreyer SJ, Boden SD. Nonoperative treatment of neck and arm pain. Spine 1998; 23:2746–54.

23. Diwan S, Manchikanti L, Benyamin RM, et al. Effectiveness of cervical epidural injections in the management of chronic neck and upper extremity pain. Pain Physician 2012;15(4):E405–34.

24. Fritz JM, Thackeray A, Brennan GP, et al. Exercise only, exercise with mechanical traction, or exercise with over-door traction for patients with cervical

radiculopathy, with or without consideration of status on a previously described subgrouping rule: a randomized clinical trial. J Orthop Sports Phys Ther 2014; 44:45–57.

25. Young IA, Michener LA, Cleland JA, et al. Manual therapy, exercise, and traction for patients with cervical radiculopathy: a randomized clinical trial. Phys Ther 2009;89:632–42.

26. Gross A, Langevin P, Burnie SJ, et al. Manipulation and mobilisation for neck pain contrasted against an inactive control or another active treatment. Cochrane Database Syst Rev 2015;9:CD004249.

27. The Back Doctor App. Apple App store and Google play store. Available at: https://apps.apple.com/us/app/back-doctor-pain-relief/id1218493415. Accessed August 10, 2020.

28. Cantu RC. Functional cervical spinal stenosis: a contraindication to participation in contact sports. Med Sci Sports Exerc 1993;25:316–7.

29. Eismont FJ, Clifford S, Goldberg M, et al. Cervical sagittal spinal canal size in spine injury. Spine 1984;9:663–6.

30. Kang JD, Figgie MP, Bohlman HH. Sagittal measurements of the cervical spine in subaxial fractures and dislocations. An analysis of two hundred and eighty-eight patients with and without neurological deficits. J Bone Joint Surg Am 1994;76: 1617–28.

31. Torg JS, Naranja RJ, Pavlov H, et al. The relationship of developmental narrowing of the cervical spinal canal to reversible and irreversible injury of the cervical spinal cord in football players. An epidemiological study. J Bone Joint Surg Am 1996;78:1308–14.

32. Torg JS, Pavlov H, Genuario SE, et al. Neuropraxia of the cervical spina cord with transient quadriplegia. J Bone Joint Surg Am 1986;68:1354–70.

33. Fay L, Huang W, Wu J, et al. Arthroplasty for cervical spondylotic myelopathy: similar results to patients with only radiculopathy at 3 years' follow-up. J Neurosurg Spine 2014;21(3):400–10.

34. Samuel AM, Moore HG, Vaishnav AS, et al. Effect of myelopathy on early clinical improvement after cervical disc replacement: a study of a local patient cohort and a large national cohort. Neurospine 2019;16(3):563–73.

35. Burneikiene S, Nelson EL, Mason A, et al. The duration of symptoms and clinical outcomes in patients undergoing anterior cervical discectomy and fusion for degenerative disc disease and radiculopathy. Spine J 2015;15:427–32.

36. Engquist M, Lofgren H, Oberg B, et al. Factors affecting the outcome of surgical versus nonsurgical treatment of cervical radiculopathy: a randomized, controlled study. Spine 2015;40:1553–63.

37. Mai HT, Chun DS, Schneider AD, et al. The difference in clinical outcomes after anterior cervical fusion, disk replacement, and foraminotomy in professional athletes. Clin Spine Surg 2018;31(1):E80–4.

38. Watkins RGIV, Chang D, Watkins RG III. Return to play after anterior cervical discectomy and fusion in professional athletes. Orthop J Sports Med 2018;6(6). 2325967118779672.

39. Burkus JK, Traynelis VC, Haid RW Jr, et al. Clinical and radiographic analysis of an artificial cervical disc: 7-year follow-up from the prestige prospective randomized controlled clinical trial. J Neurosurg Spine 2014;21:516–28.

40. Davis RJ, Nunley PD, Kim KD, et al. Two-level total disc replacement with mobi-C cervical artificial disc versus anterior discectomy and fusion: a prospective, randomized, controlled multicenter clinical trial with 4-year follow-up results. J Neurosurg Spine 2015;22:15–25.

41. Phillips FM, Geisler FH, Gilder KM, et al. Long-term outcomes of the US FDA IDE prospective, randomized controlled clinical trial comparing PCM cervical disc arthroplasty with anterior cervical discectomy and fusion. Spine 2015;40:674–83.

42. Sasso RC, Anderson PA, Riew KD, et al. Results of cervical arthroplasty compared with anterior discectomy and fusion: four- year clinical outcomes in a prospective, randomized controlled trial. J Bone Joint Surg Am 2011;93: 1684–92.

43. Hu Y, Lv G, Ren S, et al. Mid- to long-term outcomes of cervical disc arthroplasty versus anterior cervical discectomy and fusion for treatment of symptomatic cervical disc disease: a systematic review and meta-analysis of eight prospective randomized controlled trials. PLoS One 2016;11(2):e0149312.

44. Shriver MF, Lewis DJ, Kshettry VR, et al. Pseudoarthrosis rates in anterior cervical discectomy and fusion: a meta-analysis. Spine J 2015;15:2016–27.

45. Dailey A, Harrop JS, France JC. High-energy contact sports and cervical spine neuropraxia injuries: what are the criteria for return to participation? Spine 2010;35(S21):S193–201.

46. Andrews J, Jones A, Davies PR, et al. Is return to professional rugby union likely after anterior cervical spine surgery? J Bone Joint Surg Br 2008;90B:619–21.

47. Hsu WK. Outcomes following nonoperative and operative treatment for cervical disc herniations in National Football League athletes. Spine 2011;36:800–5.

48. Maroon JC, Bost JW, Petraglia AL, et al. Outcomes after anterior cervical discectomy and fusion in professional athletes. Neurosurgery 2013;73(1):103–11.

49. McAnany SJ, Overley S, Andelman S, et al. Return to play in elite contact athletes after anterior cervical discectomy and fusion: a meta-analysis. Glob Spine J 2017;7(6):552–9.

50. Chao S, Pacella MJ, Torg JS. The pathomechanics, pathophysiology and prevention of cervical spinal cord and brachial plexus injuries in athletics. Sports Med 2010;40:59–75.

51. Thomas BE, McCullen GM, Yuan HA. Cervical spine injuries in football players. J Am Acad Orthop Surg 1999;7:338–47.

52. Tempel ZJ, Bost JW, Norwig JA, et al. Significance of T2 hyperintensity on magnetic resonance imaging after cervical cord injury and return to play in professional athletes. Neurosurgery 2015;77(1):23–300.

53. Molinari RW, Pagarigan K, Dettori JR, et al. Return to play in athletes receiving cervical surgery: a symptomatic review. Glob Spine J 2016;6:89–96.

54. Brauge D, Sol JC, Djidjeli I, et al. Catastrophic return to play in rugby after double cervical arthrodesis. Clin J Sport Med 2020;30(1):e8–10.

55. Bydon M, Mathios D, Macki M, et al. Long-term patient outcomes after posterior cervical foraminotomy: an analysis of 151 cases. J Neurosurg Spine 2014;21: 727–31.

56. Skovrlj B, Gologorsky Y, Haque R, et al. Complications, outcomes, and need for fusion after minimally invasive posterior cervical foraminotomy and microdiscectomy. Spine J 2014;14:2405–11.

57. Faught RW, Church EW, Halpern CH, et al. Long-term quality of life after posterior cervical foraminotomy for radiculopathy. Clin Neurol Neurosurg 2016;142:22–5.

58. Church EW, Halpern CH, Faught RW, et al. Cervical laminoforaminotomy for radiculopathy: symptomatic and func- tional outcomes in a large cohort with long-term follow-up. Surg Neurol Int 2014;5:536.

59. Stone JL, Arnold PM, Chowdhry SA, et al. Forgotten pioneer of spinal microsurgery. Spine 2016;41:E1005–8.

60. Viezens L, Schaefer C, Beyerlein J, et al. An incomplete paraplegia following the dislocation of an artificial cervical total disc replacement: case report. J Neurosurg Spine 2013;18:255–9.

61. Niu T, Hoffman H, Lu DC. Case report: cervical artificial disc extrusion after paragliding accident. Surg Neurol Int 2017;8:138.

62. Heller JG, Sasso RC, Papadopoulos SM, et al. Comparison of BRYAN cervical disc arthroplasty with anterior cervical decompression and fusion: clinical and radiographic results of a randomized, controlled, clinical trial. Spine 2009; 34(2):101–7.

63. Mummaneni PV, Burkus JK, Haid RW, et al. Clinical and radiographic analysis of cervical disc arthroplasty compared with allograft fusion: a randomized controlled clinical trial. J Neurosurg Spine 2007;6(3):198–209.

64. Wu A, Xu H, Mullinix KP, et al. Minimum 4-year outcomes of cervical total disc arthroplasty versus fusion: a meta-analysis based on prospective randomized controlled trials. Medicine 2015;94(15):1–7.

65. Boselie TFM, Willems PC, Van Mameren H, et al. Arthroplasty versus fusion in single-level cervical degenerative disc disease. Cochrane Database Syst Rev 2015;5:CD009173.

66. Maroon JC, El-Kadi H, Abla AA, et al. Cervical neurapraxia in elite athletes: evaluation and surgical treatment. Report of five cases. J Neurosurg Spine 2007;6(4): 356–63.

67. Roberts DW, Roc GJ, Hsu WK. Outcomes of cervical and lumbar disk herniations in Major League Baseball pitchers. Orthopedics 2011;34(8):602–9.

Spinal Deformities in the Adolescent Athlete

Keith R. Bachmann, MD

KEYWORDS

- Scoliosis • Return to sport • Down syndrome • Posterior spinal fusion • Adolescents

KEY POINTS

- Scoliosis defined as lateral curvature of more than 10° is present in 2% to 3% of the population.
- Full participation in sports should be allowed and encouraged in patients with scoliosis undergoing nonoperative treatment including brace wear.
- Patients after spinal fusion can return to sport activities after discussion with their surgeon at an average interval of 6 months postsurgery depending on the activity.
- Athletes with Down syndrome have an increased risk of atlantoaxial instability and should be screened with a neutral upright lateral if they have signs or symptoms of myelopathy or cord compression.

INTRODUCTION/HISTORY/DEFINITIONS/BACKGROUND

This article focuses on sports participation among children and adolescents with spinal disorders. Sports among children is common—whether it be pickup, community, travel, school, Special Olympics, or just physical education class, children should be encouraged to remain active. During periods of rapid growth the developing spine may experience alteration in growth patterns, leading to scoliosis or kyphosis. In this chapter the authors begin by discussing screening for spinal disorders and then discuss the treatment of scoliosis including scoliosis-specific exercises, bracing, and posterior spinal fusion and the implications for sports participation. Although adolescent idiopathic scoliosis is the most common form of scoliosis, the authors also discuss sports participation among patients with other origins of scoliosis such as congenital scoliosis and scoliosis stemming from or associated with other conditions. They also touch on the cervical spine in pediatric patients with a special focus on cervical instability in Down syndrome, as it pertains to sports participation.

Adolescent idiopathic scoliosis is defined as a lateral curvature of the spine of greater than 10° measured on a posteroanterior radiograph of the spine with vertebral

Department of Orthopaedic Surgery, University of Virginia, PO Box 800159, Charlottesville, VA 22908, USA
E-mail address: kbachmann.uva@gmail.com

Clin Sports Med 40 (2021) 541–554
https://doi.org/10.1016/j.csm.2021.03.007
0278-5919/21/© 2021 Elsevier Inc. All rights reserved.

sportsmed.theclinics.com

rotation.[1] Because radiographs are a 2-dimensional image, the rotation of the spine from scoliosis rotates some of the natural curvature of the spine from the sagittal plane to the coronal plane. Only 2% to 3% of patients younger than 16 years will have a curvature of greater than 10° and only 0.3% to 0.5% will have a curve over 20°. At these small curve magnitudes patients usually present as a result of screening or incidental diagnosis not with clinical changes. The likelihood of scoliosis increases with a first-degree relative with scoliosis indicating a genetic underpinning that has not been fully elucidated and may have different sites depending on patient's ethnic background.[2]

DISCUSSION

Screening for scoliosis takes place in multiple settings: pediatrician or family medicine offices, school screenings, and the "screening" performed by families. There is evidence that the effectiveness of pediatrician screening can be improved with provider-focused interventions.[3] There is a contentious history of school screening for scoliosis with ties to an era of spinal deformity due to tuberculosis or polio bleeding into spinal deformity due to idiopathic scoliosis,[4] which has a more benign natural history.[1] Because of the relatively low incidence of scoliosis and the variable age at onset, school screening does refer some patients with scoliosis but misses some (false negatives) and generates referrals that sometimes result in radiographs but no diagnosis or treatment of scoliosis (false positives). In 1999 Yawn and colleagues reviewed a population of 2242 children screened in Rochester Minnesota and followed them to age 19 years. Screening identified 5 of the 9 children treated for scoliosis but also created referrals for 87 children who were not treated. The incidence of curves of at least 20° was 0.4%, and 448 children needed to be screened to identify one child who received treatment.[5] Karachalios and colleagues highlighted the high false-positive rate of forward bend test alone and advocated for objective data through Moire topography, humpometer, or scoliometer readings with cutoffs.[6] In a meta-analysis in 2010 Fong and colleagues noted that forward bend test alone was not sufficient for screening.[7] In 2015 Fong followed-up with a study highlighting the effectiveness of a school screening program in Hong Kong with sustained effectiveness over 5 years.[8] Altaf and colleagues[9] also discussed that screening is effective at finding scoliosis when using scoliometer or Moire topography but highlight the high referral to radiology rate of 6.6% as a hurdle to overcome.

There are also considerations of cost of school screening with Yawn and Yawn finding costs of $24.66 per child screened, $3386.25 per child with a curve of 20° or more, and $10,836 per child treated.[10] In addition to radiation and cost there is familial and patient anxiety created with a referral for scoliosis.[11] Thomas and colleagues found an increase in curve magnitude of patients presenting with scoliosis after school screening ceased in their area from 20 to 23° on average and a higher rate of patients undergoing brace and surgical treatment on presentation. There were also 48% fewer children seen from the county after school screening was discontinued.[12] As a result of these studies as well as the effectiveness of bracing demonstrated by Danielsson[13] and the BrAIST trial[14] the US Preventative Services Task Force changed the recommendation for school screening from a D in 2004 recommending against school screening to an I or insufficient rating in 2018, highlighting a lack of current evidence to balance the benefits and harms of screening.[15] They highlighted the effectiveness of bracing in limiting curve progression but cited insufficient evidence on the long-term outcomes of adolescents treated with a brace, exercises, or surgery.[16]

Diebo and colleagues[17] highlighted the lack of screening in underserved populations, and Kadhim postulated that screening underserved populations may be the solution to scoliosis school screening, highlighting a lack of referral pathway as a barrier to screening frequently cited.[18] Sports participation physicals may be an alternate avenue for screening this population. The costs of universal screening may not be viable without further evidence to support improved long-term outcomes and the difficulties associated with gathering that data, but the effectiveness of bracing at limiting curve progression should not be understated. The crux of the matter is that the same issues that limit the effectiveness of school screening—variable age at onset and variable progression after onset of scoliosis—will continue to apply. Creating multiple potential touchpoints for screening and increasing the accuracy of screening would help to identify those patients who would potentially benefit from brace wear as in **Fig. 1**.

If a patient is noted to have scoliosis this should not be a barrier to participation. There have, historically and among families, been concerns regarding lifestyle and physical activities that lead to scoliosis. Watanabe and colleagues evaluated 2600 Japanese female junior high school students aged 12 to 15 years who were due to undergo a radiographic screening after a positive screening for scoliosis and found that backpacks, time studying, playing a musical instrument, swimming, rhythmic gymnastics, artistic gymnastics, tennis, volleyball, hours of sleep and positioning during sleep, age of mother at delivery, birth weight, and maternal smoking and alcohol use were not predictive of scoliosis defined as a curvature of more than 15°. They did find

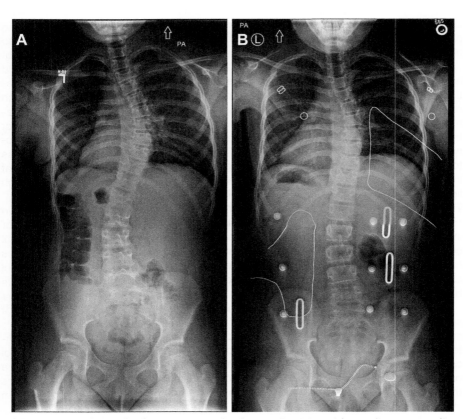

Fig. 1. (A) PA radiograph of a patient seen by their pediatrician with a scoliometer reading of 10 and thoracic Cobb angle of 40, reduced to 24 in a TLSO brace (B). PA, posteroanterior.

more frequent and earlier initiation of ballet, a mother with scoliosis, being under-weight, and dental braces were associated with increased odds of scoliosis, whereas more frequent basketball participation was protective against a diagnosis of scoli-osis.[2] Green and colleagues[19] performed a systematic review in 2009 and found that brace-treated and surgically treated patients with scoliosis can participate in sports, and nonoperative patients are encouraged to participate in sports.

Screening for scoliosis can be seen in an alternate light—rather than emphasizing the limitation of prevention of scoliosis curve progression, it can be used to encourage the normalization of scoliosis and creation of good body habits. In long-term follow-up of brace treatment with a Wilmington brace, Gabos and colleagues[20] found difficulty with functional activities of shopping, sitting, and side lying when compared with controls, and Misterska and colleagues found an increase in back and neck pain in long-term follow-up after brace treatment with a Milwaukee brace.[21] Piantoni and col-leagues[22] in 2018 found that 72% of female patients given the Brace questionnaire were psychologically affected in some way by their brace. In long-term follow-up Dan-ielsson comparing 40 patients observed with scoliosis and 37 brace-treated patients found no difference in SRS scores or SF-36 scores at a mean follow-up of 16 years after maturity.[23] Interestingly, in an earlier study out of Sweden with an earlier subset of patients comparing posterior spinal fusion with Harrington rods with brace-treated patients and normal Swedish controls, Danielsson found surgical and braced patients had slightly worse physical function on SF-36 subscales as well as worse Oswestry Disability Index. Overall, the differences were minor and the conclusion was that ad-olescents treated for scoliosis with surgery or bracing had approximately the same health-related quality of life as controls.[24]

Could these outcomes be improved with an increase in activity and improved back health created through early focus on maintenance of exercise routines and participa-tion in sport? Segreto and colleagues found patients with scoliosis being treated with a brace who participated in noncontact sports had improved functionality, self-image, expectations, and parental perception of deformity when compared with brace-treated patients who did not participate in sport.[25] This requires planning, as the typical brace wear prescription is 16 to 18 hours a day, leaving 6 to 8 hours a day for activities. In an editorial Kakar and colleagues[26] discussed decreased participation in sport after fusion as well as the osteopenia seen in patients with scoliosis, high-lighting the need for interventions to maintain activity levels in patients with scoliosis. There are more recent studies that demonstrate patients with scoliosis participating at similar levels with peers. Diarbakerli and colleagues[27] gave patients with scoliosis the international physical activity questionnaire short form and found no differences in per-centage of patients who achieved moderate activity level and sports participation compared with controls. In 2012 Negrini and colleagues[28] reviewed 607 patients and found no difference in sport participation before initiation and after 6 months of bracing with both numbers around 50%.

There is also a growing body of evidence with low-level support for scoliosis-specific exercise routines for scoliosis. Thompson and colleagues performed a systematic review of scoliosis-specific exercises compared with other nonsurgical in-terventions and found very low-quality evidence, indicating scoliosis-specific exer-cises improved function, pain, and overall health-related quality of life with no effect on self-image and mental health. They also found that bracing was more effective than scoliosis-specific exercises on measures of spinal deformity, but exercises showed greater improvements in function, health-related quality of life, self-image, mental health, and patient satisfaction.[29] A newer study not included in that review found that patients with adolescent idiopathic scoliosis (AIS) curves 12 to 20° enrolled in Schroth therapy had smaller curves than controls on average (16.3 vs 21.6, $P = .04$) and less curve progression on average (0 vs 5.6°, $P = .2$), although there was no difference in bracing at 1 year (37% vs 43%).[30] This study highlights the potential for multimodal treatment of scoliosis. Patients with a small curvature of scoliosis often want some control over their outcome, and being "observed" to watch for curve progression may not satisfy that need. Screening and giving children and families a diagnosis with no treatment may also heighten their feeling of a "disease state" of a "dangerous curve" highlighted by Linker earlier.[4] If scoliosis-specific exercises are found to be effective at prevention of progression before bracing this could fill the void. It will also highlight to patients their ability to continue to participate in activities including therapy and perhaps create better coping mechanisms as opposed to a wait and see approach. This does need to be balanced with appropriate expectations of the benefits of exercise programs. Current evidence supports bracing above all other measures for prevention of curve progression. Longer term studies are needed to see what effects, if any, scoliosis-specific exercises have on outcomes.

There are still patients who will present with large curves, likely to progress in adulthood leading to potential pulmonary restriction as well as increased likelihood of pain as an adult. The long-term Iowa studies also highlighted patient statements that they had lived a good life but wished there had been surgery as a choice when they were diagnosed.[1] For these patients the current gold standard is a posterior spinal fusion to limit longer term progression of scoliosis as in **Figs. 2** and **3**. Based on the Iowa longitudinal studies a surgical discussion takes place around 50°, especially if there is

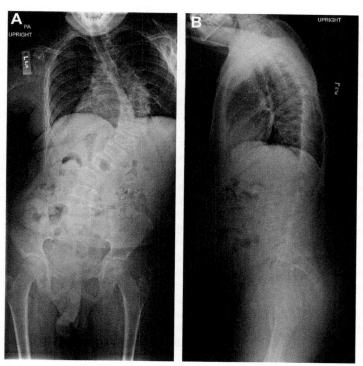

Fig. 2. PA (*A*) and lateral (*B*) upright radiographs of a patient with adolescent scoliosis preoperative.

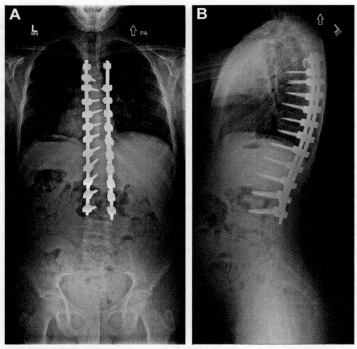

Fig. 3. PA (*A*) and lateral (*B*) upright radiographs of the patient in **Fig. 2** postoperative from posterior spinal fusion with a pedicle screw construct.

growth remaining. Fusion levels are chosen to fuse all relevant portions of the scoliotic deformity while limiting distal fusion levels to preserve segments of motion. Another group of adolescents who have not been mentioned yet is those with Scheuermann's kyphosis. The nonoperative treatment of this group is not published to the extent that patients with scoliosis is, but if they reach a deformity magnitude resulting in spine fusion the postoperative recommendations for sport will apply similarly.

The return to play for a patient after spine surgery will always be a discussion between surgeon and patient, as different surgeons will have variable timeframes for return to activity, but it is helpful to explore a framework for return to play. A survey of SRS members performed in 2002 found that formal physical therapy was unlikely to be recommended after surgery; most of the surgeons allowed patients to return to gym class and noncontact sports between 6 months and 1 year. In the same 2002 survey surgeons allowed return to contact sports after 1 year, and more than half of members who responded required or suggested that their patients not return to collision sports ever. This survey included surgery for scoliosis, kyphosis, and spondylolisthesis and was done in an era of mostly segmental, but not pedicle screw fixation.[31] Lehman and colleagues therefore conducted a survey in 2015 of members of the Spinal Deformity Study Group with different clinical case scenarios involving different construct types (hooks, pedicle screws, hybrid) as well as different lowest instrumented vertebra. They found that with pedicle screw instrumentation the barriers to return to sport were lowered with surgeons allowing return to running by 3 months, contact and noncontact sports by 6 months, and collision sports by 12 months. There was still a propensity to not allow return to collision sports, with 20% of respondents never allowing return to collision sports, and the overall rate increased with a lower distal fusion level with 33% of surgeons not allowing return to collision sports when the lowest instrumented vertebra was L4. Only one surgeon had anecdotal information about a failure of instrumentation due to pullout or implant failure in a patient who went snowboarding 2 weeks post-op.[32]

Although patients appreciate the advice of their treating surgeon, it is also important to look at what patients actually do in regard to return to school, play, and sport. Fabricant in 2012 looked at return to athletic activity in 42 athletically active adolescents who underwent posterior spinal fusion for idiopathic scoliosis. At average follow-up of 5.5 years, 25 patients had returned to sports at an equal or higher level of physical activity. The main reason cited among patients who did not return to the same level of sport was lack of flexibility followed by back pain, deconditioning, loss of desire, and scheduling. Predictors of inability to return to same level of sport were lowest instrumented vertebra, Lenke 5 or 6 curves, and final SRS score.[33] In 2014 a prospective study out of Ireland examined the timing and predictors of return to short-term functional activity after posterior spinal fusion in patients with adolescent idiopathic scoliosis. They followed-up 77 patients for up to 2 years or until full resumption of activities. They found the median time to return to school full time was 10 weeks, with the majority (77.5%) returning by 16 weeks. About 94.6% had returned by 24 weeks, and all patients had returned to school by 36 weeks postoperative. They found that preoperative curves greater than 70°, postoperative weight loss greater than 5 kg, and minor perioperative respiratory complications predicted delayed return to school. They also examined return to unrestricted physical activity. At 24 weeks 51.4% of patients had returned to unrestricted activities and 88.5% had returned by 1 year postoperative. Only 3 subjects reported nonreturn to unrestricted activity at final follow-up of 2 years.[34] Recently Sarwahi and colleagues validated a patient questionnaire survey about return to athletics. They validated the survey in 75 patients and then gave the validated survey to 95 respondents. They had 6.4% of patients return to school in less than a month, 71% between 1 and 3 months, 18% took 4 to 6 months, and the final 4.3% somewhere between 7 months and 1 year. Higher body mass index and Cobb greater than 70° correlated with later return to school. On the other end of the spectrum of 64 patients who participated in sports pre-op, 82% of patients returned to sport by 6 months and 33% of them had returned at 3 months. They note that these rates of return were faster than they recommended but they did not note any implant failure or loss of correction that they could correlate with return to sport at 2-year follow-up.[35]

There are recent motion analysis studies evaluating the return to sportlike activities among patients after spinal fusion for adolescent idiopathic scoliosis. Kakar and colleagues evaluated 10 patients who were physically active minimum 1 year postoperative from spinal fusion and 10 age-matched controls. The spinal fusion patients ran at a self-selected speed perceived to be hard. The control patients then ran at a matched speed, and spine and lower extremity kinematics were recorded with a 3-dimensional motion capture system. The spinal fusion patients exhibited greater lower trunk defined as L1-L5 and pelvis segmental axial rotation during running. The spinal fusion patients also exhibited less ankle plantar flexion.[36] The same group a year earlier examined spine kinematics during stop jump: an activity with a run up, single leg jump landing with 2 feet to then perform a vertical leap off of 2 feet. Posterior spinal fusion patients were paired with controls. Overall, there were small sometimes not statistically significant differences in the various phases of the stop jump, but the investigators found similar kinematics between the 2 groups when performing this complex task.[37] Some of this ability to maintain function may be explained by the increased motion that is distributed to unfused segments as demonstrated by Marks and colleagues. In their study more distal fusion levels resulted in increased motion at the remaining motion levels on lateral bending radiographs but not on forward bend.[38] This change in spinal motion after spinal fusion underpins the excitement and embracing of nonfusion surgical treatment of scoliosis with anterior spinal tether and posterior ratcheting systems recently obtaining humanitarian device exemptions through the Food and Drug Administration but there is a paucity of follow-up and motion data to provide any insight other than speculation on their effects on sports participation.

What should a surgeon do with this information when crafting a return to sport plan? Sarwahi noted that motivated patients interested in sport will likely find their way back to sport. There is also some humbling that occurs, as patients will not always follow a surgeon's advice. If there is a strong reason or support for restrictions then patient education needs to be crafted to relay that to patients. Otherwise relying on the strong 3-column fixation that can be provided by pedicle screw fixation and then providing guidelines for patient expectations is appropriate. From the studies presented and the American Academy of Orthopedic Surgeons' OrthoInfo Website as well as the SRS AIS surgery FAQs there are rough guidelines that can be presented to patients:

- No heavy lifting or repetitive bending for the first 6 weeks
- Encourage walking for the first 6 weeks
- Backpacks and lifting up to 10 pounds allowed after 6 weeks, most lifting restrictions removed at 3 months after surgery
- Return to school at 4 to 6 weeks while ensuring availability of a home schooling or tutoring program
- Return to more vigorous training for sport and progression to sports beginning at 3 months after surgery at the discretion of the treating surgeon regarding specific milestones for return and limitations[39,40]

There is a paucity of published information on patients with other causes of their scoliosis and participation in sport. Most spinal deformity is now treated with pedicle screw instrumentation regardless of cause, so there is likely room for participation in sport depending on the cause of the deformity.

Congenital Scoliosis and Kyphosis

Depending on the involvement of the scoliosis and the treatment pursued encouragement of activity should be considered as noted earlier. At times these deformities are complex and involve broad segments of the thoracic or lumbar spine. Even before any surgical fusion these patients may have complex fusion masses. A careful neurologic examination should be obtained, and radiographs should be scrutinized for any congenital kyphosis especially at the cervicothoracic junction and the thoracolumbar junction. Because of the association of neural axis abnormalities these patients typically undergo MRI of their entire spine and so the clinician will be armed with more information about any presence of stenosis and can counsel the patient regarding any sport avoidance; this may include steering patients away from collision sports or sports with a high risk for axial load especially through the neck such as cheerleading or gymnastics and football. The physical examination should be monitored at follow-up and stability of the spine around the congenitally different segments of the spine assumed to be normal unless imaging predicts otherwise. Special attention should be paid to congenital fusions in the remainder of the spinal column including the cervical spine. These patients also have associations with congenital heart and renal abnormalities as well as the aforementioned neural axis abnormalities, so careful consideration of the entire patient and involvement of other specialists are needed.

Syndromic Scoliosis

Marfan syndrome can present with an idiopathic-like scoliosis due to an underlying collagen disorder as well as possible dural ectasia, vascular, and ocular involvement. This is another patient population where close consultation and consideration of the entirety of the patient may trump the spine involvement alone. After spinal fusion the hypermobility should be considered when counseling patients on return to sport.

Neurofibromatosis patients can have dystrophic or more typical longer segment scoliosis. They often have neurofibromas involving their spine and dural ectasia. These patients frequently have poor bone quality and erosion due to dural ectasia, leading to narrow posterior elements and possible loss of the anterior column of the spine as in **Fig. 4**. The decision to return to sport will depend on many patient-specific factors and should involve a discussion with the family regarding their risks while attempting to allow for as much activity as possible, as these patients are typically ambulatory and want to participate if able.

Chiari malformation patients typically undergo occipital decompression at the direction of neurosurgery, and consultation between services should be undertaken to determine the patient's ability to return to sports at varying levels. Their scoliosis is idiopathic-like and is treated as such from a surgical perspective if needed.

Syringomyelia frequently is associated with Chiari malformation, tethered cord, or another alteration of cerebrospinal fluid flow. Consultation with a neurosurgical service and close discussion with the patient and family before return to activities likely without collision or contact and minimizing axial load.

Scoliosis associated with dwarfism will depend on the various forms of dwarfism, as some are associated with spinal stenosis and others may present with other skeletal abnormalities that will limit sports participation.

Neuromuscular Scoliosis

Patients with cerebral palsy may participate in adapted sports leagues as well as enjoy adapted swimming, equine therapy, or sporting activities with their families such as

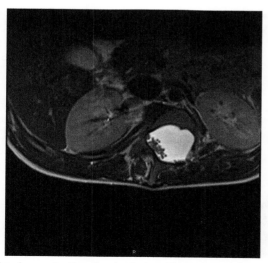

Fig. 4. Axial MRI slice demonstrating dural ectasia with erosion of the pedicles and anterior vertebral body in a patient with neurofibromatosis.

inner tubing. A discussion should be had with the family about activities that the patient participates in and risks especially for proximal junction kyphosis of a typical T2-pelvis fusion with activities. Frequently spinal fusion allows for increased postural stability and a return to recreational activities.

Duchenne muscular dystrophy scoliosis fusions are typically undertaken at the time the patient becomes wheelchair dependent, but an attempt should be made with the patient and family to encourage continued participation as able.

This is by no means an exhaustive list of all conditions with associated scoliosis but highlights many of the decisions for return to sport a pediatric spine provider may be faced with. The value of shared decision-making with the patient and family is notable in these patient populations with a goal of maintaining or resuming participation for these patient populations, understanding the stability of the construct that is achieved with pedicle screw instrumentation.

The cervical spine in Down syndrome receives attention from the American Academy of Pediatrics in their health supervision guidelines with screening for atlantoaxial instability recommended. They note in the guidelines that screening for asymptomatic children is not supported but participation in collision sports and sports such as gymnastics and trampoline in older children may carry extra risk and that participation in Special Olympics may require additional screening.[41] The forms for Special Olympics ask thoroughly about signs of myelopathy or cord compression such as bowel and bladder dysfunction, ataxia, spasticity, or numbness and tingling of the upper extremities. If these signs are not present the athlete does not require radiographic screening as in **Fig. 5**.[42] In a recent article Bouchard and colleagues presented a new algorithm after reviewing 88 flexion-extension cervical spine series and found only one patient who did not have abnormalities on a neutral upright lateral that had abnormal values on a flexion-extension series, and this patient did not have any signs or symptoms of myelopathy or cord compression and was observed.[43] The screening and participation of this group and other patients in Special Olympics activities that are noncollision sports should hinge on the physical examination with supporting image studies as needed.

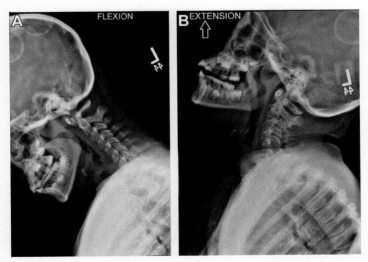

Fig. 5. Flexion (A) and extension (B) lateral radiographs of a patient with Down syndrome demonstrating an increase in atlantodental interval in flexion to 6 mm.

Other chapters in this text present concepts that may also apply to children: prevention of spine injuries; evaluation of spinal injuries for any patient older than 10 years should be similar whether on field or involving transient quadriparesis or cervical neuropraxia. Evaluation of low back pain in adolescent athletes is more likely to uncover spondylolysis than disc herniation, but treatment of the subsequent diagnosis can be undertaken similar to the pathways described in the other articles of this issue.

SUMMARY

Idiopathic scoliosis will be noted in 2% to 3% of typically developing athletes. Sports physicals are an opportunity to screen for spinal deformity and to promote healthy involvement in activities. Bracing is effective at limiting further progression if a curve progresses beyond 20°. If spinal fusion is performed most surgeons allow return to noncontact and contact sports by 6 to 12 months. There are many other conditions associated with scoliosis that require a more nuanced approach and assessment of the entire patient. Patients with Down syndrome should be examined for myelopathy before participation and a lateral radiograph obtained if concerned for instability.

CLINICS CARE POINTS

- Scoliosis defined as lateral curvature on radiographs of more than 10 degrees is present in 2% to 3% of the population.
- Full participation in sports should be allowed and encouraged in patients with scoliosis undergoing nonoperative treatment including brace wear.
- Patients after spinal fusion can return to sport activities after discussion with their surgeon at an average interval of 6 months postsurgery depending on the activity.
- Athletes with Down syndrome have an increased risk of atlantoaxial instability and should be screened with a neutral upright lateral if they have signs or symptoms of myelopathy or cord compression.

DISCLOSURE

K.R. Bachmann—consulting with DePuy Synthes Spine.

REFERENCES

1. Weinstein SL. The natural history of adolescent idiopathic scoliosis. J Pediatr Orthop 2019;39(6):S44–6.
2. Watanabe K, Michikawa T, Yonezawa I, et al. Physical activities and lifestyle factors related to adolescent idiopathic scoliosis. J Bone Joint Surg Am 2017;99(4): 284–94.
3. Diaz MCG, Wysocki T, Crutchfield JH, et al. Provider-focused intervention to promote comprehensive screening for adolescent idiopathic scoliosis by primary care pediatricians. Am J Med Qual 2019;34(2):182–8.
4. Linker B. The role of history in America's scoliosis screening programs. Am J Public Health 2012;102(4):606–16.
5. Yawn BP, Yawn RA, Hodge D, et al. A population-based study of school scoliosis screening. J Am Med Assoc 1999;282(15):1427–32.
6. Karachalios T, Sofianos J, Roidis N, et al. Ten-year follow-up evaluation of a school screening program for scoliosis: Is the forward-bending test an accurate

diagnostic criterion for the screening of scoliosis? Spine (Phila Pa 1976) 1999; 24(22):2318–24.

7. Fong DYT, Lee CF, Cheung KMC, et al. A meta-analysis of the clinical effectiveness of school scoliosis screening. Spine (Phila Pa 1976) 2010;35(10):1061–71.

8. Fong DYT, Cheung KMC, Wong YW, et al. A population-based cohort study of 394,401 children followed for 10 years exhibits sustained effectiveness of scoliosis screening. Spine J 2015;15(5):825–33.

9. Altaf F, Drinkwater J, Phan K, et al. Systematic review of school scoliosis screening. Spine Deform 2017;5(5):303–9.

10. Yawn BP, Yawn RA. The estimated cost of school scoliosis screening. Spine (Phila Pa 1976) 2000;25(18):2387–91.

11. Hines T, Roland S, Nguyen D, et al. School Scoliosis Screenings. Spine (Phila Pa 1976) 2015;40(21):E1135–43.

12. Thomas JJ, Stans AA, Milbrandt TA, et al. Does school screening affect scoliosis curve magnitude at presentation to a pediatric orthopedic clinic? Spine Deform 2018;6(4):403–8.

13. Danielsson AJ, Hasserius R, Ohlin A, et al. A prospective study of brace treatment versus observation alone in adolescent idiopathic scoliosis: a follow-up mean of 16 years after maturity. Spine (Phila Pa 1976) 2007;32(20):2198–207.

14. Weinstein SL, Dolan LA, Wright JG, et al. Effects of bracing in adolescents with idiopathic scoliosis. N Engl J Med 2013;369(16):1512–21.

15. Grossman DC, Curry SJ, Owens DK, et al. Screening for adolescent Idiopathic Scoliosis US preventive services task force recommendation statement. JAMA 2018;319(2):165–72.

16. Dunn J, Henrikson NB, Morrison CC, et al. Screening for adolescent idiopathic scoliosis evidence report and systematic review for the US preventive services task force. JAMA 2018;319(2):173–87.

17. Diebo BG, Segreto FA, Solow M, et al. Adolescent idiopathic scoliosis care in an underserved inner-city population: screening, bracing, and patient- and parent-reported outcomes. Spine Deform 2019;7(4):559–64.

18. Kadhim M, Lucak T, Schexnayder S, et al. Current status of scoliosis school screening: targeted screening of underserved populations may be the solution. Public Health 2020;178:72–7.

19. Green BN, Johnson C, Moreau W. Is physical activity contraindicated for individuals with scoliosis? A systematic literature review. J Chiropr Med 2009;8(1): 25–37.

20. Gabos PG, Bojescul JA, Bowen JR, et al. Long-term follow-up of female patients with idiopathic scoliosis treated with the Wilmington orthosis. J Bone Joint Surg Am 2004;86(9):1891–9.

21. Misterska E, Głowacki J, Okręt A, et al. Back and neck pain and function in females with adolescent idiopathic scoliosis: a follow-up at least 23 years after conservative treatment with a Milwaukee brace. PLoS One 2017;12(12):1–18.

22. Piantoni L, Tello CA, Remondino RG, et al. Quality of life and patient satisfaction in bracing treatment of adolescent idiopathic scoliosis. Scoliosis Spinal Disord 2018;13(1):1–12.

23. Danielsson AJ, Hasserius R, Ohlin A, et al. Health-related quality of life in untreated versus brace-treated patients with adolescent idiopathic scoliosis. Spine (Phila Pa 1976) 2010;35(2):199–205.

24. Danielsson AJ, Wiklund I, Pehrsson K, et al. Health-related quality of life in patients with adolescent idiopathic scoliosis: a matched follow-up at least 20 years after treatment with brace or surgery. Eur Spine J 2001;10(4):278–88.

25. Segreto FA, Messina JC, Doran JP, et al. Noncontact sports participation in adolescent idiopathic scoliosis: Effects on parent-reported and patient-reported outcomes. J Pediatr Orthop B 2019;28(4):356–61.

26. Kakar RS, Simpson KJ, DAS BM, et al. Review of physical activity benefits and potential considerations for individuals with surgical fusion of spine for scoliosis. Int J Exerc Sci 2017;10(2):166–77.

27. Diarbakerli E, Grauers A, Möller H, et al. Adolescents with and without idiopathic scoliosis have similar self-reported level of physical activity: a cross-sectional study. Scoliosis Spinal Disord 2016;11(1):1–7.

28. Negrini S, Donzelli S, Negrini F, et al. Bracing does not change the sport habits of patients. Stud Health Technol Inform 2012;176:437–40.

29. Thompson JY, Williamson EM, Williams MA, et al. Effectiveness of scoliosis-specific exercises for adolescent idiopathic scoliosis compared with other non-surgical interventions: a systematic review and meta-analysis. Physiotherapy 2019;105:214–34.

30. Zapata KA, Sucato DJ, Jo CH. Physical therapy scoliosis-specific exercises may reduce curve progression in mild adolescent idiopathic scoliosis curves. Pediatr Phys Ther 2019;31(3):280–5.

31. Rubery PT, Bradford DS. Athletic activity after spine surgery in children and adolescents: Results of a survey. Spine (Phila Pa 1976) 2002;27(4):423–7.

32. Lehman RA, Kang DG, Lenke LG, et al. Return to sports after surgery to correct adolescent idiopathic scoliosis: a survey of the Spinal Deformity Study Group. Spine J [Internet] 2015;15(5):951–8.

33. Fabricant PD, Admoni SH, Green DW, et al. Return to athletic activity after posterior spinal fusion for adolescent idiopathic scoliosis: analysis of independent predictors. J Pediatr Orthop 2012;32(3):259–65.

34. Tarrant RC, O'Loughlin PF, Lynch S, et al. Timing and predictors of return to short-term functional activity in adolescent idiopathic scoliosis after posterior spinal fusion: a prospective study. Spine (Phila Pa 1976) 2014;39(18):1471–8.

35. Sarwahi V, Wendolowski S, Gecelter R, et al. When do patients return to physical activities and athletics after scoliosis surgery? A validated patient questionnaire based study. Spine (Phila Pa 1976) 2018;43(3):167–71.

36. Kakar RS, Li Y, Brown CN, et al. Spine and lower extremity kinematics exhibited during running by adolescent idiopathic scoliosis patients with spinal fusion. Spine Deform [Internet] 2019;7(2):254–61.

37. Kakar RS, Li Y, Brown CN, et al. Spine kinematics exhibited during the stop-jump by physically active individuals with adolescent idiopathic scoliosis and spinal fusion. Spine J 2018;18(1):155–63.

38. Marks M, Newton PO, Petcharaporn M, et al. Postoperative segmental motion of the unfused spine distal to the fusion in 100 patients with adolescent idiopathic scoliosis. Spine (Phila Pa 1976) 2012;37(10):826–32.

39. Society SR. Surgery for adolescent idiopathic scoliosis: FAQ [Internet]. Available at: https://www.srs.org/patients-and-families/common-questions-and-glossary/ais-surgery-faqs. Accessed August 28, 2020.

40. OrthoInfo. Surgical treatment for scoliosis [Internet]. Available at: https://orthoinfo.aaos.org/en/treatment/surgical-treatment-for-scoliosis/. Accessed August 28, 2020.

41. Bull MJ, Saal HM, Braddock SR, et al. Clinical report - health supervision for children with down syndrome. Pediatrics 2011;128:393–406.

42. Special Olympics athlete Registration form [Internet]. Available at: https://www.specialolympicsva.org/get-involved/athlete-resources. Accessed August 29, 2020.

43. Bouchard M, Bauer JM, Bompadre V, et al. An updated algorithm for radiographic screening of upper cervical instability in patients with down syndrome. Spine Deform 2019;7(6):950–6.

Return to Play for Cervical and Lumbar Spine Conditions

George W. Fryhofer, MD, MTR, Harvey E. Smith, MD*

KEYWORDS

- Return to play • Spinal cord injury • Sports • Athlete • Cervical spine
- Lumbar spine

KEY POINTS

- Return to play guidelines and expectations for cervical and lumbar spinal conditions do exist, but the implementation of these guidelines in clinical practice often is a subjective process driven by surgeon experience.
- In general, return to play requires that an athlete has painless active range of motion, painless sport-specific exercise, and full strength without neurologic deficit.
- A variety of special circumstances may complicate the decision to return to play, and this decision must be made in a case-specific and patient-specific manner.

INTRODUCTION

Return to play (RTP) readily is discussed in the context of recovery from injuries sustained while playing a sport; however, a majority of spinal cord injuries (SCIs) and conditions in the general population are unrelated to sports.[1] Therefore, RTP guidelines— although important for professional athletics—also are useful in the treatment of patients who may not be professional athletes but who also wish to return to their preferred recreational activities.

Unfortunately, despite decades of study, universal guidelines for the management of cervical and lumbar spine conditions and returning to sports still are lacking and, in the absence of randomized controlled trials, are driven mostly by case reports, case series, reviews, and expert opinion. In general, expert opinion recommendations for RTP require that an athlete has painless active range of motion, painless sport-specific exercise, and full strength without neurologic deficit.

This article reviews the most common cervical and lumbar spine conditions encountered among professional and recreational athletes as well as the associated RTP guidelines and expectations for each condition.

Department of Orthopaedic Surgery, University of Pennsylvania School of Medicine, 3737 Market Street, 6th Floor, Philadelphia, PA 19104, USA
* Corresponding author.
E-mail address: harvey.smith@pennmedicine.upenn.edu

Clin Sports Med 40 (2021) 555–569
https://doi.org/10.1016/j.csm.2021.04.002
0278-5919/21/© 2021 Elsevier Inc. All rights reserved.

CERVICAL SPINE

The incidence of SCI in the United States is 54 cases per 1 million people, which equates to approximately 17,810 new SCI cases each year.[1] Since 2015, the leading causes of SCIs have been vehicular accidents (38.6%), falls (32.3%), violence (14.0%), and sports (7.8%).[1]

Axial loading is the most common mechanism resulting in catastrophic sports-related cervical spine injuries. These injuries usually arise following a head-down collision, such as might result from spearing in American football, where the tackler leads with the crown of the helmet—banned since 1976. Similarly, the spear tackle in rugby, in which a player is lifted up and then dropped on the ground to land on the back, head, or neck, also has been banned due to its association with spinal injury. Despite the banning of such high-risk maneuvers in contact sports, however, cervical spine injuries still occur.

To better understand the epidemiology and outcomes of cervical spine injury and sports, previous research has focused on American football, given its popularity in the United States as a high-contact/collision sport. As of 2019, approximately 74,000 student-athletes participated in National Collegiate Athletic Association (NCAA) football,[2] with an additional approximately 1700 athletes playing each year at the professional level in the National Football League (NFL). Over an 11-year period in the NFL from 2000 to 2010, more than 2200 injuries were identified involving the spine or axial skeleton, equating to approximately 200 injuries per season.[3]

The incidence of any spine injury among NFL players is approximately 0.93 injuries per 1000 athlete-exposures (AEs),[3] and the rate of cervical spine injury alone is approximately 0.42 injuries per 1000 AEs. Compared with professional football players, the rate of cervical spine injury among college players is similar (approximately 0.48 per 1000 AEs); however, the rate of injury at the high school level is approximately 2-times to 5-times lower.[4,5] Among high school athletes, cervical spine injury is most common among football players, followed by wrestling and girls' gymnastics.[4]

Among athletes in the NCAA, true cervical spine injuries only represent approximately 10% of all reported neck and cervical spine injuries, and 60% of athletes with reported neck injury are able to RTP within 24 hours of injury.[6] Regarding RTP, several groups have proposed guidelines specific to the type of cervical spine injury,[7–9] and a survey of members of the Cervical Spine Research Society (CSRS)[10] (**Box 1**) provides a recent update to these recommendations, all of which are discussed later. General contraindications to RTP that are not necessarily related to prior trauma are listed in **Box 2**.

In addition to the above, Maroon and Bailes[11] have classified patients with cervical spine injuries further into 1 of 3 types: type 1—permanent SCI; type 2—transient SCI; and type 3—radiologic abnormality without neurologic deficit. They recommend that patients with type 1 injuries should never RTP; patients with type 2 injuries may be allowed to RTP if a complete work-up is negative without neurologic deficit; and patients with type 3 injuries may be allowed to RTP as long as radiographic findings do not suggest instability (such as spear tackler spine).

Although these RTP guidelines are helpful, their implementation in clinical practice often is a subjective process driven more by external factors, such as surgeon experience; and, in some cases, published guidelines may play little to no role in the decision for a given patient to RTP.[12,13] Nevertheless, in the following sections, the authors do their best to summarize the available RTP guidelines and expectations for each of the most common cervical spine conditions found in sports.

Box 1

Summary of recommendations for return to play after cervical spine injury with strong or unanimous consensus from the Cervical Spine Research Society survey (Schroeder and colleagues, 2020)

Cervical stenosis

Following an episode of transient paralysis, asymptomatic athletes with NO T2-signal change and a spinal canal diameter greater than 10 mm are allowed to RTP, but those with a canal diameter less than 10 mm should be taken on a case-by-case basis.

Following an episode of transient paralysis, asymptomatic athletes with RESOLVED T2-signal changes and a spinal canal diameter greater than 13 mm are allowed to RTP; those with a canal diameter between 10 mm and 13 mm should be considered on a case-by-case basis, and those with a canal diameter less than 10 mm should not RTP.

Cervical trauma and/or surgery in collision athletes

Asymptomatic athletes with NO T2-signal change after a solid 1-level/2-level ACDF are allowed to RTP, but those after 3-level ACDF should not RTP.

Asymptomatic athletes with CONTINUED T2-signal change after a solid 2-level/3-level ACDF should not RTP, but those after 1-level ACDF should be taken on a case-by-case basis.

Asymptomatic athletes with a solid fusion after a compression fracture, burst fracture, or facet fracture with no instability and no T2-signal change are allowed to RTP.

Following an episode of transient paralysis, asymptomatic athletes with NO T2-signal change following a 1-level/2-level ACDF are allowed to RTP but following a corpectomy or posterior cervical surgery RTP should be taken on a case-by-case basis.

General considerations

Athletes with prior nonoperative or operative treatment of cervical spinal pathology (with the exception of a stinger) should undergo a screening MRI prior to playing competitive collision/contact sports.

Athletes who are asymptomatic for less than 5 min following a stinger are allowed to RTP, but for those with symptoms lasting greater than 5 min, RTP should be taken on a case-by-case basis.

Stingers and Burners

Stingers, also known as burners, describe brachial plexus injuries that usually are transient, most commonly involving the upper trunk. Originally thought to be caused by stretch of the brachial plexus when a player's shoulder is forced laterally with the

Box 2

General contraindications to athletic participation not necessarily related to prior trauma (Cantu and colleagues; Vaccaro and colleagues)

Arnold-Chiari malformation

Multiple-level Klippel-Feil deformity

Ankylosing spondylitis

Diffuse idiopathic skeletal hyperostosis

Symptomatic cervical disc herniation

Status post–cervical laminectomy

Status post–3-level cervical fusion

neck and head tilted in the other direction (ie, a traction injury from falling onto or tackling with the shoulder),[14] it later was found that direct compression of the most superficial portion of the brachial plexus at Erb point by the superomedial scapula (ie, direct blow to the shoulder pads) is the more common mechanism of injury.[15] A third potential mechanism of injury is due to neuroforaminal nerve root compression during hyperextension of the cervical spine.[16] Stingers most commonly involve the exiting C5 and C6 nerve roots, with symptoms ranging from mild paresthesias and weakness to transient arm monoplegia.[7] Symptoms usually last for a few seconds to minutes but in some cases may last up to several weeks.[9] Younger patients and those experiencing a stinger for the first time with transient symptoms are more likely to have sustained trauma to the brachial plexus alone, whereas symptoms in an older player with a history of recurrent stingers—termed, *chronic burner syndrome*—also may be due to cervical nerve root compression at the neural foramen.[17]

Treatment of stingers is nonoperative, and patients are recommended to refrain from athletics while symptoms still are present. In reviews by Torg and Ramsey-Emrhein[8] and by Cantu and colleagues,[7] RTP is allowed for neurologically intact patients with 1 or 2 stinger episodes lasting less than 24 hours and full cervical range of motion.[7] In the recent survey of CSRS members, there also was a strong consensus that patients with stinger symptoms lasting less than 5 minutes be allowed to RTP.[10] A relative contraindication to RTP is having a stinger with symptoms lasting for more than 24 hours or having 3 or more stinger episodes.[7] For cases of stinger symptoms persisting beyond 2 weeks, Weinstein[18] recommends obtaining electrodiagnostic studies. The presence of moderate fibrillation potentials on electrodiagnostics or mild fibrillation potentials with clinical weakness is a contraindication to RTP.

Cervical Strain

Cervical strain or sprain is not uncommon, accounting for 6.9% of all injuries among NFL players[3] and 1% of all injuries among National Basketball Association (NBA) players.[19]

Although cervical strain may seem relatively benign, the possibility of occult instability must be ruled out. At a minimum, flexion-extension radiographs of the cervical spine should be obtained initially and at 2 weeks to 4 weeks after injury.[16] Rigid cervical collar immobilization is recommended if instability is suspected. Magnetic resonance imaging (MRI) evaluation is indicated if range of motion is significantly limited or if radicular symptoms are present.

In order to RTP after cervical strain, a patient must be asymptomatic with full painless range of motion of the cervial spine, full strength, and pain-free sport-specific exercise.[16,20]

Cervical Stenosis and Cervical Cord Neuropraxia (Transient Quadriplegia/Paresis)

Transient quadriplegia, or cervical cord neuropraxia, can occur following a hyperextension injury and presents as burning paresthesias with or without motor weakness that last anywhere from 10 minutes to 15 minutes to up to 36 hours. The incidence of cord neuropraxia in college athletes is approximately 0.13 per 1000 AEs.[21] To better understand the relationship between cervical stenosis and cervical SCI, Torg and colleagues[22] developed the Torg ratio—that is, the width of the spinal canal divided by the width of the vertebral body—which could help to identify congenital cervical canal stenosis (if ratio <0.80) and was 93% sensitive for predicting transient neuropraxia. Specificity of the Torg ratio is poor, however, with a low positive predictive value (0.2%), which limits its usefulness as a screening tool.[22,23]

Similar to that of burners and stingers, treatment of cervical cord neuropraxia usually is nonoperative; however, persistent symptoms or cord signal abnormality may warrant surgical decompression. In reviews by Torg and Ramsey-Emrhein[8] and Cantu and colleagues,[7] there was no contraindication to RTP for patients who had only 1 episode of transient quadriparesis with symptoms lasting less than 24 hours and had complete recovery,[7] even with a canal/vertebral body ratio of 0.8 or less.[8] A relative contraindication to RTP was transient quadriparesis lasting more than 24 hours.[7] Absolute contraindications to RTP following transient quadriparesis included any residual neck discomfort, reduced range of motion, abnormal neurologic examination, cord signal abnormality, functional stenosis (ie, loss of cerebrospinal fluid around cord)[23] on computed tomography and MRI, a stenotic canal with anteroposterior diameter less than 13 mm, a single neuropraxia episode lasting more than 36 hours, or multiple episodes.[7,8]

In the recent survey of CSRS members, the spinal canal diameter criterion contraindicating RTP following transient paralysis was clarified.[10] There was a strong consensus that if there was no T2 signal change on MRI, then RTP with canal diameter greater than 10 mm (as opposed to 13 mm) should be allowed RTP. Additionally, patients with resolved T2 signal changes after transient paralysis and spinal canal diameter less than 13 mm should not be allowed to RTP.

Cervical Disc Herniation

The rates of cervical disc disease and cervical disc herniation are suspected to be higher among contact athletes compared with the general population.[24] Among NFL players, disc-related pathology accounts for only 5.8% and 28% of cervical spine and lumbar spine injuries and yet is responsible for one of the greatest mean sports participation days lost by injury type, second only to frank SCI.[3] The most common levels affected in the cervical spine of NFL players are C3-4, C4-5, and C5-6, and players with a cervical disc herniation are out of play an average of 3 months.[25] Although some investigators have suggested that participation in noncontact sports actually may protect against disc herniation, a previous case-control study of patients in the general population identified no significant risk of harm or protective benefit between participation in sporting activity and sustaining a cervical or lumbar disc herniation (LDH).[26]

Unfortunately, cervical disc herniations among professional athletes can be career altering. A study of how preexisting cervical spine pathology has an impact on the careers of NFL players demonstrated that players with cervical disc herniation were significantly less likely to get drafted compared with those without disc herniation (48.1% vs 78.1%, respectively).[27] For those who were drafted with disc herniation, however, there was no difference in years or games played or in player performance score compared with those without spine pathology.

RTP following nonoperative and/or surgical treatment of cervical disc pathology has been studied in several case series,[27–35] and Kang and colleagues[36] provide a nice summary. Rates of RTP were higher for surgical treatment with anterior cervical discectomy and fusion (ACDF) in 2 of 3 studies that included a nonoperative treatment arm.[30,33,34] Rates of RTP for surgical treatment generally ranged from 66% to 88%,[28,30,31,33,34] although 100% RTP was observed in 2 studies with smaller sample size.[29,32] RTP was not without complication, however, with some patients experiencing career-ending recurrent disc herniation,[32] new spinal contusion,[29] or recurrent symptoms[28] after returning. Saigal and colleagues[35] found that RTP was significantly higher among noninstrumented cervical spine patients compared with those with instrumentation (97% vs 72%, respectively); however, this study included all types of cervical spine pathology and was not limited specifically to cases of cervical disc herniation.

Torg and Ramsey-Emrhein[8] and Cantu and colleagues[7] recommend RTP for patients who have recovered from single-level ACDF with intact neurologic status and have only occasional stiffness or pain.[7] Relative contraindications to RTP are healed 1-level or 2-level anterior or posterior cervical fusions.[7] An absolute contraindication to RTP is cervical laminectomy or 3-level anterior or posterior cervical fusion.[7] There also is a strong consensus among CSRS members that "asymptomatic athletes with no T2-signal change after a solid 1-level/2-level ACDF are allowed to RTP, but a 3-level ACDF should not RTP."[10]

Cervical Fracture or Instability

Cervical fracture is one of least common types of spinal injury seen in athletics but when it occurs is found most often in collision sports. In a study of NFL players over an 11-year period, fractures accounted for only 1.8% (n = 18) of all cervical spine injuries yet were responsible for more time out of play than all other cervical injuries, with an average of 120 playing days lost.[3] Cervical fractures also occur in other collision sports, such as hockey, where a registry study of Canadian players identified 188 cervical spine fractures and/or dislocations from 1943 to 2005.[37]

Possible fracture patterns include spinous process fractures, Jefferson fractures (ie, fracture of the anterior and posterior C1 arch), compression fractures, chance fractures (ie, flexion-distraction injuries involving the anterior, middle, and posterior spinal columns), or burst fractures with or without multicolumn involvement.[24]

Treatment depends on fracture stability and neurologic status. Unstable fractures generally necessitate surgical fixation, whereas stable fracture patterns may be treated successfully with cervical collar immobilization. RTP can be considered only after the fracture is fully healed and no sooner than 8 weeks to 10 weeks after injury.[24] In the evaluation for RTP, at the very least, flexion-extension radiographs of the cervical spine must be obtained to assess for instability, and patients must have full pain-free range of motion without neurologic deficit. An MRI also is recommended prior to return to contact or collision sports.[10]

In reviews by Torg and Ramsey-Emrhein[8] and Cantu and colleagues,[7] RTP is allowed for healed C1 or C2 fractures with normal range of motion and for healed subaxial fractures without sagittal pane deformity.[7] RTP also is allowed for an asymptomatic clay shoveler (C7 spinous process) fracture.[9] Furthermore, there is strong consensus from members of the CSRS that "asymptomatic athletes with a solid fusion after a compression fracture, burst fracture, or facet fracture with no instability and no T2-signal change are allowed to RTP."[10] Absolute contraindications to RTP include a history of C1-2 fusion, C1-2 hypermobility with anterior dens interval of 4 mm or greater, any posttraumatic or ligamentous kyphotic deformity or subaxial instability (>11° angulation or >3.5-mm translation), or spear tackler spine—that is, loss of cervical lordosis with evidence of prior bony or ligamentous injury.[7]

LUMBAR SPINE

Approximately 10% to 15% of all athletes complain of low back pain.[38] This number can vary significantly among sports, however, with 1 study of college soccer players in Japan reporting a lifetime incidence of low back pain as high as 76.6%.[39]

Among injuries sustained to the axial skeleton during athletics, the predilection for lumbosacral (vs cervical or thoracic) spine involvement varies widely among professional sports, with lower rates of lumbosacral involvement observed for hockey (4.8%)[37] and football (30.9%)[3] players and the highest rates observed among NBA players (86.6%).[19] In the study of NBA players, even with axial and nonaxial injuries pooled together, lumbar strain still was the third most frequent injury overall, occurring in 7.9% of players.[19] The rate of lumbar injury among competitive adolescent soccer players is lower, however, with lumbar spine injuries accounting for only 3% of all injuries sustained over the course of 5 seasons in a study of more than 12,000 athletes.[40] Of all lumbar spine injuries in that population, the most common diagnoses were low back pain (49.4%), lumbar strain (15.2%), and spondylolysis (3.9%), with spondylolisthesis (1.6%), and fracture (1.3%) less common.[40]

For general RTP, and in cases of lumbar fracture, spondylolysis, spondylolisthesis, or disc herniation, Ball and colleagues[41] again recommend resolution of symptoms, full lumbar spine range of motion, and absence of pain while performing sport-specific exercises.

Lumbar Strain

Approximately 70% of all cases of low back pain in the general population can be attributed to lumbar strain.[42] Among athletes, a study of adolescent soccer players over 5 seasons found injuries in the lumbar region (44.5%) to be the most common, followed by the erector spinae (11.9%) and quadratus lumborum (5.8%), with injury to the multifidi (0.6%) being relatively rare.[40]

In their review of RTP in lumbar spine conditions, Eck and Riley[43] recommend that lumbar strain be treated conservatively, with RTP allowed after the patient has regained full range of motion in order to prevent further injury. They also emphasize the importance of therapy to break the cycle of pain and muscle imbalance—wherein an initial painful injury can lead to muscle disuse and imbalance, which then predisposes to additional injury, continued pain, and further weakness. Patients may RTP once this cycle is broken and rehabilitation is complete.

Lumbar Disc Degeneration

The etiologies of lumbar disc degeneration (LDD) are multiple, including disc desiccation, inflammation, changes in the microbiome, disc acidity, axial overloading, and genetic predisposition.[44]

The rate of LDD among athletes depends on the sport. A cross-sectional study of 308 university athletes in Japan found significantly higher odds of degenerative disc findings on MRI among baseball players (59.7%) and swimmers (57.5%)—but not for other sports—compared with nonathletes (31.4%), with the L5-S1 and L4-5 levels the most commonly affected.[39] Among NBA players, LDD accounts for only 0.9% of all injuries but 3.6% of total games missed.[19]

First-line treatment of low back pain due to isolated LDD is conservative, but, if nonoperative measures fail, then surgical options may include lumbar fusion or total lumbar disc replacement (TDR). Data regarding outcomes of fusion for treatment of isolated LDD among athletes are limited and there is a lack of consensus regarding the efficacy of fusion for axial low back pain. Unlike fusion, TDR for treatment of isolated LDD has been studied in both athletes[45] and active-duty military personnel,[46] with 94.9% and 83% of patients, respectively, returning to sports or unrestricted full duty. In both studies, a majority of patients had returned to sports or to unrestricted full duty by 6 months postoperatively. Among athletes after TDR, minimum RTP recommendations for noncontact sports are no sooner than 3 months and contact sports no sooner than 4 months to 6 months after surgery.[45] Among military personnel after TDR, return to activity is recommended to begin with nonimpact training at 3 months, light impact training by 4 to 5 months, and unrestricted full duty by 6 months after surgery.[46]

Lumbar Disc Herniation

In contrast to isolated LDD, LDH has been well studied among athletes. In a retrospective study of NFL players over 12 seasons, LDH accounted for 28% of lumbar spine injuries, with 74% involving the lumbar spine, most commonly at the L5-S1 and L4-5 levels.[25] Initial treatment of LDH typically is nonoperative, although the Spine Patient Outcomes Research Trial studies and others have reported good outcomes following surgical treatment of LDH.[47–50] It is unclear, however, whether the findings of these randomized controlled studies of patients in the general population can be extrapolated to a cohort of high-performance athletes seeking to return to sports.

Retrospective cohort studies among athletes have shown that although surgery not always is performed in the treatment of LDH, the average rate of RTP following single-level lumbar discectomy ranges from 80% to 90%.[51–54] In 1 study, 50% of patients had returned to play by 3 months, 72% by 6 months, and 84% by 12 months, and RTP timing was not related to the anatomic level of the neurologic deficit.[51] In patients who do RTP, future career length also has been shown to be negatively impacted by player age following LDH, with older players with LDH having shorter postinjury careers.[52]

With regard to which treatment is most effective—surgical versus nonoperative—a systematic review found no difference in the rate of RTP following surgical versus nonoperative treatment of LDH.[55] That review also noted that although not described in all studies, the rate of a patient's return to prior level of sport function following microdiscectomy—38% to 65%—was lower than the overall rate of RTP, meaning that just because a patient is able to RTP does not mean that they necessarily will be able to go back to playing at the same level as they were preinjury.[55] Using sports statistics, an athlete's postinjury performance following lumbar discectomy has been calculated to range from 64.4% to 103.6% of the athlete's preinjury baseline.[56] In another study, type of sport also has been found to affect RTP following surgical treatment of LDH, with MLB players having higher rates of RTP and NFL players have lower rates of RTP compared with athletes in other sports.[52] Among MLB players alone, patients who had surgery had shorter careers on average compared with patients treated nonoperatively.[52]

In another study of MLB players (and in contrast to the systematic review by Reiman and colleagues,[55] discussed previously), surgical treatment of LDH has been associated with delayed RTP compared with nonoperative treatment (8.7 months vs 3.6 months, respectively), which was an effect that did vary according to player position, with hitters and infielders benefitting the most from nonoperative treatment.[57] Additionally, in another study, NBA players, patients who underwent surgery had decreased rates of RTP compared with controls (75% vs 88%, respectively) and fewer games played the following season. The players in that study who were able to RTP, however, following surgery ultimately regained athletic performance similar to preinjury levels,[58] although in other cases a "full recovery" may not be evident until the second or third season postinjury.[59]

RTP criteria for LDH are generalized regardless of surgical versus nonoperative treatment. These include symptom resolution, full pain-free lumbar range of motion, and pain-free sport-specific exercise.

Thoracolumbar Fractures

In the 3-column model of acute thoracolumbar spinal injuries, Denis[60] divides fractures into minor (transverse process, facet, pars interarticularis, and spinous process) and major (compression, burst, seat belt–type, and fracture-dislocation) injury subtypes. Minor injuries tend to be stable with lower-energy mechanisms that affect the lower lumbar region, whereas major injuries are more unstable with higher-energy mechanisms that tend to occur higher up at the thoracolumbar junction.[61] It has been suggested that a majority of lumbar fractures sustained during sports participation are minor injuries with 1-column involvement that usually can be treated nonoperatively.[41]

In a study of adolescent soccer players, fracture accounted for only 1.3% of all lumbar spine injuries sustained over a 5-season period but was associated with the greatest delay in RTP with a median recovery period of approximately 5 months.[40] For thoracolumbar fractures treated nonoperatively, there are reports of patients managed with thoracolumbar spinal orthosis, with successful RTP after 3 months.[62,63]

RTP criteria for thoracolumbar fracture are generalized, including symptom resolution, full pain-free lumbar range of motion, fracture healing, and pain-free sport-specific exercise.

Lumbar Spondylolysis and Isthmic Spondylolisthesis

Lumbar spondylolysis is a discontinuity of the pars interarticularis and can be either unilateral or bilateral. Evidence of spondylolysis is found in 6% of the general population[64] but is more common among athletes, affecting 47% of adolescent athletes presenting with low back pain in 1 study[65] and 44% of young hockey players presenting with low back pain in another study.[66]

Lumbar spondylolysis also has been classically described for sports like gymnastics, where repetitive hyperextension caused by movements, such as back walkovers and vaults, may predispose to injury. In 1 study, bilateral L5 pars defects were identified by radiograph in 11% of healthy competitive female gymnasts.[67] The investigators of that study noted that despite being asymptomatic at the time of study evaluation, 3 of the gymnasts included in the study previously had sought medical attention for low back pain and had radiographs that initially were negative, which suggests that spondylolysis can develop in a patient that continues to train despite pain.[67] In addition to the repetitive flexion/extension movements that put gymnasts at risk for injury, a study of hockey players found that 73% of spondylolysis occurred on the player's shooting side, which highlights the role of repetitive forceful directional rotation as another possible mechanism of injury.[66] Spondylolysis usually presents as back pain that is exacerbated by spinal extension rather than flexion and, unless other injuries are present, is not associated with neurologic deficit.[41]

Lumbar isthmic spondylolisthesis refers to displacement of lumbar vertebrae anteriorly with respect to the vertebrae below it in the setting of bilateral pars discontinuity (ie, bilateral spondylolysis). Spondylolysis and isthmic spondylolisthesis exist as a continuum of disease, and athletes with bilateral spondylolysis are at risk for developing spondylolisthesis.

RTP in cases of lumbar spondylolysis with or without isthmic spondylolisthesis depends on whether nonoperative versus operative treatment is pursued. For isolated spondylolysis or for low-grade spondylolisthesis, first-line treatment usually is nonoperative.

Longitudinal cohort and retrospective studies describing nonoperative treatment of athletes with symptomatic lumbar spondylolysis and spondylolisthesis have demonstrated 70% to 91% good to excellent long-term outcomes and high rates of RTP without surgery or fusion and a low likelihood of spondylolisthesis progression if the initial slip was less than 30%.[68–70] EL Rassi and colleagues[71] showed that patients who returned to athletics prior to the recommended 3-month rest period were more symptomatic with only 8% "excellent" functional results compared with 97%

"excellent" results in patients who did adhere to the 3-month rest period. Despite differences in patient-reported outcomes, duration of activity cessation had no effect on healing, with 100% radiographic union observed in both groups.[71]

In general, the RTP protocols utilized in most clinical studies of nonoperative treatment recommend sport cessation for at least 3 months to 6 months,[69,71–73] followed by rehabilitation and gradual return to sport-specific exercise,[68,74] although some investigators have proposed RTP with a nonrigid brace by as early as 2 months to 3 months if the patient remains pain-free during sport-specific activity.[68] Some investigators also are more stringent with the type of athletic activity allowed, with Eck and Riley[43] allowing noncontact sports at 12 months but recommending against return to contact sports at any time.

Nonoperative treatment not always is successful, however, and surgical treatment is recommended after at least 9 months to 12 months of persistent symptoms despite conservative treatment[68] or for high-grade (>50%) slips that may be concerning for slip progression.[75] Surgical options include direct repair of the pars defects alone (for slips up to 3 mm with a normal disc) or lumbar fusion with or without instrumentation.[70] Lumbar fusion techniques include anterior lumbar interbody fusion, posterior lumbar interbody fusion, and posterolateral fusion, with posterolateral fusion providing less consistent results.[76,77] In addition to posterior approaches, anterior interbody fusion is another option that has been associated with decreased morbidity but similar patient outcomes for single-level fusions.[78]

In 2002, Rubery and colleagues[79] performed a survey of 261 members of the Scoliosis Research Society (SRS) in order to identify surgeon preferences for return to athletic activity following surgical treatment of scoliosis or spondylolisthesis. For slips less than 50%, most surgeons supported withholding return to noncontact sports for 6 months and withholding return to contact sports for 1 year, with more than 50% of surgeons also requiring or suggesting that patients with high-grade slips never return to collision sports. Solid radiographic fusion on patient follow-up is preferred, with 80% to 90% of SRS survey respondents indicating that radiographic appearance after surgery impacted the RTP decision either "moderately" or a "great deal."[79] Similarly, Radcliff and colleagues[70] recommend return to sport no sooner than 6 months to 12 months after surgery. Their review also describes a structured rehabilitation program starting 2 weeks after surgery, with gradual progression from nonimpact aerobic activity at 2 weeks to 4 weeks with the spine in neutral alignment, then advancing to introduction of impact and dynamic exercises at 3 months, and concluding with sport-specific exercises between 4 months and 6 months.[70]

Adolescent Idiopathic Scoliosis

Adolescent idiopathic scoliosis (AIS) is defined as a coronal curve measured by Cobb technique to be greater than 10° in children 10 years old to 16 years old. AIS is present in 2% to 3% of the adolescent population, although fewer than 10% of patients with AIS actually require surgery.[80] Many of these young patients are active and involved in athletics prior to surgery, and RTP is an important consideration.

Fabricant and colleagues[81] performed a retrospective cohort study to identify patient factors predictive of RTP in 42 athletically active adolescents with AIS who underwent posterior spinal fusion. In that study, the rate of RTP was 59.5%, defined as returning to sports at an equal or higher level of physical activity compared with preoperative baseline. There was a stepwise decrease in RTP associated with successively lower distal fusion levels, with 100% RTP observed for constructs ending at T11 but only 20% RTP for fusion constructs extending down to L4. Patients with lower number Lenke curve types (eg, thoracic curves) and higher SRS-22 scores also had higher rates of

RTP. Criteria for RTP were (1) pain-free range of motion and (2) no radiographic signs of curve progression or hardware migration (3) no sooner than 4 months after surgery, and the average time for full clearance for RTP was 7.4 months. The investigators warn, however, against over-interpretation of their findings and note that although the study represents 1 center's experience that may prove useful in counseling patients, it is not meant to provide strict guidelines or supplant surgeon discretion.

A 2002 survey of members of the SRS also was conducted to identify surgeon preferences and trends regarding RTP after scoliosis fusion.[79] More than 50% of surgeons in that study would allow noncontact sports after 6 months and contact sports after 1 year, with 60% of surgeons recommending against or expressly forbidding collision sports (wrestling, football, hockey, and gymnastics) at any time after scoliosis fusion. Time from surgery and use of instrumentation were the most significant self-reported factors influencing a surgeon's decision to allow athletic activity after surgery, and distal fusion level mattered only slightly or not at all for just over half of the surgeons who responded to the survey.

SUMMARY

Although the safety of contact sports has improved over the years, participation in any sport always carries a risk of injury. When cervical or lumbar spine injuries do occur, prompt diagnosis is essential, and athletes must be held out of the sport if indicated to prevent further harm and allow for recovery. In these cases, RTP expectations and guidelines are useful both for counseling patients who wish to return to their pre-injury way of life as soon as possible and for guiding a physician's treatment decisions. General requirements for RTP include resolution of symptoms without neurologic deficit, full pain-free range of motion, and pain-free sport-specific exercise. There are a variety of special circumstances, however, that may complicate RTP, and, as such, the decision to RTP must be made in a case-specific and patient-specific manner, and published guidelines should not necessarily supplant surgeon discretion.

CLINICS CARE POINTS

- Approximately 60% of college athletes with reported neck injury are able to RTP within 24 hours of injury.
- Athletes with prior nonoperative or operative treatment of cervical spinal pathology (with the exception of a stinger) should undergo a screening MRI prior to playing competitive collision/contact sports.
- Symptomatic cervical disc herniation is a general contraindication to athletic participation.
- Athletes who are asymptomatic within 5 min following a stinger are allowed to RTP, but for those with symptoms lasting greater than 5 min, RTP should be taken on a case-by-case basis.
- RTP after lumbar spine injury generally requires resolution of symptoms, full lumbar spine range of motion, and absence of pain while performing sport-specific exercises.
- The majority of surgeons recommend that patients with high-grade spondylolisthesis with slips greater than 50% should never return to collision sports.
- Among patients with adolescent idiopathic scoliosis who have undergone posterior spinal fusion, there is a stepwise decrease in RTP associated with successively lower distal fusion levels, with 100% RTP observed for constructs ending at T11, but only 20% RTP for fusion constructs extending down to L4.
- The decision to RTP must be made in a case-specific and patient-specific manner, and published guidelines should not necessarily supplant surgeon discretion.

DISCLOSURE

The authors have nothing to disclose.

REFERENCES

1. NSCISC. National spinal cord injury statistical center (facts and figures at a glance). Birmingham, AL: University of Alabama at Birmingham; 2020.
2. Irick E. NCAA sports sponsorship and participation rates report 1981-82 – 2018-19. Indianapolis, IN: National Collegiate Athletic Association; 2019.
3. Mall NA, Buchowski J, Zebala L, et al. Spine and Axial Skeleton Injuries in the National Football League. Am J Sports Med 2012;40(8):1755–61.
4. Meron A, McMullen C, Laker SR, et al. Epidemiology of cervical spine injuries in high school athletes over a ten-year period. PM R 2018;10(4):365–72.
5. Shankar PR, Fields SK, Collins CL, et al. Epidemiology of High School and Collegiate Football Injuries in the United States, 2005-2006. Am J Sports Med 2007; 35(8):1295–303.
6. Deckey DG, Makovicka JL, Chung AS, et al. Neck and Cervical Spine Injuries in National College Athletic Association Athletes. Spine 2020;45(1):55–64.
7. Cantu RC, Li YM, Abdulhamid M, et al. Return to play after cervical spine injury in sports. Curr Sports Med Rep 2013;12(1):14–7.
8. Torg JS, Ramsey-Emrhein JA. Cervical Spine and brachial plexus injuries: return-to-play recommendations. Phys Sportsmed 1997;25(7):61–88.
9. Vaccaro AR, Klein GR, Ciccoti M, et al. Return to play criteria for the athlete with cervical spine injuries resulting in stinger and transient quadriplegia/paresis. Spine J 2002;2(5):351–6.
10. Schroeder GD, Canseco JA, Patel PD, et al. Updated return-to-play recommendations for collision athletes after cervical spine injury: a modified Delphi consensus study with the cervical spine research society. Neurosurgery 2020; 87(4):647–54.
11. Maroon JC, Bailes JE. Athletes with cervical spine injury. Spine (Phila Pa 1976) 1996;21(19):2294–9.
12. Morganti C, Sweeney CA, Albanese SA, et al. Return to play after cervical spine injury. Spine 2001;26(10):1131–6.
13. Ukogu C, Bienstock D, Ferrer C, et al. Physician decision-making in return to play after cervical spine injury. Clin Spine Surg A Spine 2020;33(7):e330–6.
14. Bateman JE. Nerve injuries about the shoulder in sports. J Bone Joint Surg Am 1967;49(4):785–92.
15. Markey KL, Di Benedetto M, Curl WW. Upper trunk brachial plexopathy. Am J Sports Med 1993;21(5):650–5.
16. Huang P, Anissipour A, McGee W, et al. Return-to-play recommendations after cervical, thoracic, and lumbar spine injuries. Sports Health 2016;8(1):19–25.
17. Levitz CL, Reilly PJ, Torg JS. The pathomechanics of chronic, recurrent cervical nerve root neurapraxia. Am J Sports Med 1997;25(1):73–6.
18. Weinstein SM. Assessment and rehabilitation of an athlete with a "stinger": a model for the management of noncatastrophic athletic cervical spine injury. Clin Sports Med 1998;17(1):127–35.
19. Drakos MC, Domb B, Starkey C, et al. Injury in the National Basketball Association. Sports Health 2010;2(4):284–90.
20. Torg JS. Cervical spine injuries and the return to football. Sports Health 2009;1(5): 376–83.

21. Torg JS, Pavlov H, Genuario SE, et al. Neurapraxia of the cervical spinal cord with transient quadriplegia. J Bone Joint Surg Am 1986;68(9):1354–70.

22. Torg JS, Naranja RJ, Pavlov H, et al. The relationship of developmental narrowing of the cervical spinal canal to reversible and irreversible injury of the cervical spinal cord in football players. An Epidemiological Study. J Bone Joint Surg 1996; 78(9):1308–14.

23. Herzog RJ, Wiens JJ, Dillingham MF, et al. Normal cervical spine morphometry and cervical spinal stenosis in asymptomatic professional football players. Spine 1991;16(Supplement):S178–86.

24. Paulus S, Kennedy DJ. Return to play considerations for cervical spine injuries in athletes. Phys Med Rehabil Clin N Am 2014;25(4):723–33.

25. Gray BL, Buchowski JM, Bumpass DB, et al. Disc herniations in the national football league. Spine 2013;38(22):1934–8.

26. Mundt DJ, Kelsey JL, Golden AL, et al. An epidemiologic study of sports and weight lifting as possible risk factors for herniated lumbar and cervical discs. The Northeast Collaborative Group on Low Back Pain. Am J Sports Med 1993; 21(6):854–60.

27. Schroeder GD, Lynch TS, Gibbs DB, et al. The impact of a cervical spine diagnosis on the careers of National Football League Athletes. Spine 2014;39(12): 947–52.

28. Andrews J, Jones A, Davies PR, et al. Is return to professional rugby union likely after anterior cervical spinal surgery? J Bone Joint Surg Br 2008;90(5):619–21.

29. Brigham CD, Capo J. Cervical Spinal Cord Contusion in Professional Athletes. Spine (Phila Pa 1976) 2013;38(4):315–23.

30. Hsu WK. Outcomes following nonoperative and operative treatment for cervical disc herniations in National Football League Athletes. Spine (Phila Pa 1976) 2011;36(10):800–5.

31. Maroon JC, Bost JW, Petraglia AL, et al. Outcomes after anterior cervical discectomy and fusion in professional athletes. Neurosurgery 2013;73(1):103–12 [discussion 112].

32. Maroon JC, El-Kadi H, Abla AA, et al. Cervical neurapraxia in elite athletes: evaluation and surgical treatment. Report of five cases. J Neurosurg Spine 2007;6(4): 356–63.

33. Meredith DS, Jones KJ, Barnes R, et al. Operative and nonoperative treatment of cervical disc herniation in National Football League Athletes. Am J Sports Med 2013;41(9):2054–8.

34. Roberts DW, Roc GJ, Hsu WK. Outcomes of cervical and lumbar disk herniations in Major League Baseball pitchers. Orthopedics 2011;34(8):602–9.

35. Saigal R, Batjer HH, Ellenbogen RG, et al. Return to play for neurosurgical patients. World Neurosurg 2014;82(3–4):485–91.

36. Kang DG, Anderson JC, Lehman RA Jr. Return to play after cervical disc surgery. Clin Sports Med 2016;35(4):529–43.

37. Tator CH, Provvidenza C, Cassidy JD. Spinal injuries in Canadian ice hockey: an update to 2005. Clin J Sport Med 2009;19(6):451–6.

38. De Luigi AJ. Low back pain in the adolescent athlete. Phys Med Rehabil Clin N Am 2014;25(4):763–88.

39. Hangai M, Kaneoka K, Hinotsu S, et al. Lumbar intervertebral disk degeneration in athletes. Am J Sports Med 2009;37(1):149–55.

40. Shah T, Cloke DJ, Rushton S, et al. Lower Back Symptoms in Adolescent Soccer Players: Predictors of Functional Recovery. Orthop J Sports Med 2014;2(4). 2325967114529703.

41. Ball JR, Harris CB, Lee J, et al. Lumbar spine injuries in sports: review of the literature and current treatment recommendations. Sports Med Open 2019;5(1):26.
42. Hart LG, Deyo RA, Cherkin DC. Physician office visits for low back pain. Spine 1995;20(1):11–9.
43. Eck JC, Riley LH 3rd. Return to play after lumbar spine conditions and surgeries. Clin Sports Med 2004;23(3):367–79, viii.
44. Amin RM, Andrade NS, Neuman BJ. Lumbar disc herniation. Curr Rev Musculoskelet Med 2017;10(4):507–16.
45. Siepe CJ, Wiechert K, Khattab MF, et al. Total lumbar disc replacement in athletes: clinical results, return to sport and athletic performance. Eur Spine J 2007;16(7):1001–13.
46. Tumialan LM, Ponton RP, Garvin A, et al. Arthroplasty in the military: a preliminary experience with ProDisc-C and ProDisc-L. Neurosurg Focus 2010;28(5):E18.
47. Buttermann GR. The effect of spinal steroid injections for degenerative disc disease. Spine J 2004;4(5):495–505.
48. Peul WC, Van Houwelingen HC, Van Den Hout WB, et al. Surgery versus prolonged conservative treatment for sciatica. N Engl J Med 2007;356(22):2245–56.
49. Weinstein JN, Lurie JD, Tosteson TD, et al. Surgical vs nonoperative treatment for lumbar disk Herniation. JAMA 2006;296(20):2451.
50. Weinstein JN, Tosteson TD, Lurie JD, et al. Surgical vs nonoperative treatment for lumbar disk Herniation. JAMA 2006;296(20):2441.
51. Watkins RG, Hanna R, Chang D, et al. Return-to-play outcomes after microscopic lumbar diskectomy in professional athletes. Am J Sports Med 2012;40(11):2530–5.
52. Hsu WK, McCarthy KJ, Savage JW, et al. The Professional Athlete Spine Initiative: outcomes after lumbar disc herniation in 342 elite professional athletes. Spine J 2011;11(3):180–6.
53. Savage JW, Hsu WK. Statistical Performance in National Football League Athletes After Lumbar Discectomy. Clin J Sport Med 2010;20(5):350–4.
54. Weistroffer JK, Hsu WK. Return-to-play rates in national football league linemen after treatment for lumbar disk herniation. Am J Sports Med 2011;39(3):632–6.
55. Reiman MP, Sylvain J, Loudon JK, et al. Return to sport after open and microdiscectomy surgery versus conservative treatment for lumbar disc herniation: a systematic review with meta-analysis. Br J Sports Med 2016;50(4):221–30.
56. Nair R, Kahlenberg CA, Hsu WK. Outcomes of lumbar discectomy in elite athletes: the need for high-level evidence. Clin Orthop Relat Res 2015;473(6):1971–7.
57. Earhart JS, Roberts D, Roc G, et al. Effects of lumbar disk herniation on the careers of professional baseball players. Orthopedics 2012;35(1):43–9.
58. Anakwenze OA, Namdari S, Auerbach JD, et al. Athletic performance outcomes following lumbar discectomy in professional basketball players. Spine (Phila Pa 1976) 2010;35(7):825–8.
59. Minhas SV, Kester BS, Larkin KE, et al. The Effect of an Orthopaedic Surgical Procedure in the National Basketball Association. Am J Sports Med 2016;44(4):1056–61.
60. Denis F. The three column spine and its significance in the classification of acute thoracolumbar spinal injuries. Spine (Phila Pa 1976) 1983;8(8):817–31.
61. Wood KB, Li W, Lebl DR, et al. Management of thoracolumbar spine fractures. Spine J 2014;14(1):145–64.
62. McHugh-Pierzina VL, Zillmer DA, Giangarra CE. Thoracic compression fracture in a basketball player. J Athl Train 1995;30(2):163–4.

63. Elattrache N, Fadale PD, Fu FH. Thoracic spine fracture in a football player: a case report. Am J Sports Med 1993;21(1):157–60.
64. Fredrickson BE, Baker D, McHolick WJ, et al. The natural history of spondylolysis and spondylolisthesis. J Bone Joibt Surg Am 1984;66(5):699–707.
65. Micheli LJ. Back pain in young athletes. Arch Pediatr Adolesc Med 1995; 149(1):15.
66. Donaldson LD. Spondylolysis in elite junior-level ice hockey players. Sports Health 2014;6(4):356–9.
67. Jackson DW, Wiltse LL, Cirincoine RJ. Spondylolysis in the female gymnast. Clin Orthop Relat Res 1976;117:68–73.
68. Miller SF, Congeni J, Swanson K. Long-term functional and anatomical follow-up of early detected spondylolysis in young athletes. Am J Sports Med 2004;32(4): 928–33.
69. Morita T, Ikata T, Katoh S, et al. Lumbar spondylolysis in children and adolescents. J Bone Joint Surg Br 1995;77(4):620–5.
70. Radcliff KE, Kalantar SB, Reitman CA. Surgical management of spondylolysis and spondylolisthesis in athletes: indications and return to play. Curr Sports Med Rep 2009;8(1):35–40.
71. El Rassi G, Takemitsu M, Woratanarat P, et al. Lumbar spondylolysis in pediatric and adolescent soccer players. Am J Sports Med 2005;33(11):1688–93.
72. Standaert CJ, Herring SA. Expert opinion and controversies in sports and musculoskeletal medicine: the diagnosis and treatment of spondylolysis in adolescent athletes. Arch Phys Med Rehabil 2007;88(4):537–40.
73. Kurd MF, Patel D, Norton R, et al. Nonoperative treatment of symptomatic spondylolysis. J Spinal Disord Tech 2007;20(8):560–4.
74. d'Hemecourt PA, Zurakowski D, Kriemler S, et al. Spondylolysis: returning the athlete to sports participation with brace treatment. Orthopedics 2002;25(6): 653–7.
75. Transfeldt EE, Mehbod AA. Evidence-based medicine analysis of isthmic spondylolisthesis treatment including reduction versus fusion in situ for high-grade slips. Spine (Phila Pa 1976) 2007;32(19 Suppl):S126–9.
76. Müslüman AM, Yılmaz A, Cansever T, et al. Posterior lumbar interbody fusion versus posterolateral fusion with instrumentation in the treatment of low-grade isthmic spondylolisthesis: midterm clinical outcomes. J Neurosurg Spine 2011; 14(4):488–96.
77. Madan S, Boeree NR. Outcome of posterior lumbar interbody fusion versus posterolateral fusion for spondylolytic spondylolisthesis. Spine (Phila Pa 1976) 2002;27(14):1536–42.
78. Pradhan BB, Nassar JA, Delamarter RB, et al. Single-level lumbar spine fusion: a comparison of anterior and posterior approaches. J Spinal Disord Tech 2002; 15(5):355–61.
79. Rubery PT, Bradford DS. Athletic activity after spine surgery in children and adolescents. Spine 2002;27(4):423–7.
80. Lonstein JE. Scoliosis. Clin Orthop Rel Res 2006;443:248–59.
81. Fabricant PD, Admoni S-H, Green DW, et al. Return to athletic activity after posterior spinal fusion for adolescent idiopathic scoliosis. J Pediatr Orthop 2012; 32(3):259–65.

Spinal Care in the Aging Athlete

Pramod N. Kamalapathy, BA, Hamid Hassanzadeh, MD*

KEYWORDS

- Athlete • Osteoporosis • Management • Spinal stenosis
- Degenerative disk disease • Facet join arthritis • Spondylolysis/spondylolisthesis

KEY POINTS

- Watch out for warning signs that may appear in disease presentations and adjust workouts as necessary.
- Patient education is crucial to prevent reinjury and help manage expectations.
- Exercise has shown to outweigh consequences of increased activity and disk degeneration due to age.

INTRODUCTION

The older generation is staying more active than before. The term aging athlete is a large and growing group, denoting anyone from 35 to 90 years old. This group faces adversities from increased activity; however, they also experience age-related health issues, such as spinal stenosis, osteoporosis complicated by fragility fractures, and degenerative disk disease. Exercise provides a variety of benefits: from increased bone health to decreased risk of common comorbidities. Nevertheless, this comes at a cost for increasing risk for injury from exercising and activity as they can also experience typical sports injuries. Ultimately, exercise has shown to outweigh the consequences of increasing activity and disk degeneration that can develop in middle-aged adults.

LOW BACK PAIN

Low back pain is one of the most common benign conditions in athletes, especially older athletes, affecting 50% to 80% of adults during their lifetime.[1] As people age, sarcopenia and osteopenia are 2 of the most common causes of lower back pain. Muscle mass peaks in the fifth decade and gradually declines by 1% to 2% per year.[2] Muscle atrophy occurs due to decline in number and area of muscle fibers.

Department of Orthopaedics, University of Virginia, 400 Ray Hunt C. Drive, Charlottesville, VA 22903, USA
* Corresponding author.
E-mail address: Hh4xd@virginia.edu

Clin Sports Med 40 (2021) 571–584
https://doi.org/10.1016/j.csm.2021.04.003
0278-5919/21/© 2021 Elsevier Inc. All rights reserved.

sportsmed.theclinics.com

The strength of the muscle fibers will occur first, reducing flexibility, structure, and balance. Contrarily, bone mass peaks at the third decade, following age-related decline. Many theories exist surrounding aging and why decline occurs, such as accumulation of DNA damage, age-related mutation or deletion of mitochondrial DNA, or reduction in androgynous concentration (in men).[3–5] Primarily, there are 2 processes that affect aging of the spine: degenerative changes and reduction in bone mass. The etiologies of low back pain are wide: degenerative disk disease, osteoarthropathy, lumbar stenosis, and osteoporosis, and we discuss these further in this article.

OSTEOPOROSIS
Introduction

Osteoporosis is a skeletal disease characterized by decreased bone mass and alteration in bone structure, which increases fracture risk.[6] The World Health Organization defines osteoporosis as bone mineral density (BMD) T score less than −2.5, and low bone mass as T score between −1.0 and −2.5.[7] The prevalence for osteoporosis is estimated at approximately 11% for adults aged 50 years or older overall (16.5% prevalence in woman and 5.1% in men).[8] The elderly population accounts for most of the disease burden, with 70% of all fractures sustained by those aged at least 65 years.[9] The prevalence of osteoporosis is increasing as the number of elderly patients continues to increase. Cost of care for osteoporosis has increased more than 118% over 15 years, nearly $50 billion over more than a decade.[8]

Risk Factors

The pathogenesis of osteoporosis is multimodal, involving various factors such as demographics, nutrition, social factors, genetics, and physical and hormonal changes. **Table 1** summarizes the risk factors discussed in the following.

Demographics

Some nonmodifiable risk factors include older age, gender, ethnic background, and prior fractures.[6,10–12] The prevalence of osteoporosis in men older than 60 was 3 times higher than those aged 50 to 59.[13] Certain populations have an increased rate of

Table 1 Osteoporosis risk factors	
Modifiable risk factors	
Alcohol	Poor nutrition
Smoking	Stress
Low body mass index	Insufficient exercise
Major nonmodifiable risk factors	
Old age	Gender (female)
History of falls	Prior fracture
Ethnicity	Family history of osteoporosis
Secondary causes of osteoporosis	
Hypogonadism	Vitamin D deficiency
Hyperparathyroidism	Renal disease
Chronic liver disease	Cardiovascular disease
Diabetes mellitus	Iatrogenic

osteoporosis. Hispanic individuals have a higher rate of fracture at the spine, and Caucasian individuals have an increased rate at the femoral neck.[14,15]

Social factors

Physical exercise and activity stimulate bone health and growth.[6,16] Nicotine, smoking, and alcohol are related to osteoporotic fracture risk by inhibiting osteoblast production, resulting in cell death.[17]

Nutritional deficiency

Many nutrients, such as vitamins (A, B, C, E, K), minerals, and macronutrients such as protein and fats increase bone health.[18] Therefore, it is essential to maintain healthy life choices, as drinking excess amounts of alcohol can impair bone formation. The Framingham Osteoporosis Study assessed dietary patterns to better understand and counsel the public on nutrition. They highlighted that processed foods present with significantly lower femoral neck BMD than the low-fat milk group. For men, fruit and vegetables, and cereal groups had the greatest BMD at all bone sites, and candy was the lowest for both genders.[19]

Genetics

Individuals with lower BMD can have different fracture risk, highlighting the polygenic nature of fracture risk and osteoporosis.[20] Low BMD, fracture risk, and biomechanical bone structure have all been associated with genes and single nucleotide polymorphisms.[20] In 2018, Morris and colleagues[21] identified 301 novel significant loci that potentially explain approximately 20% of genetic variation. Future research studies should be conducted to determine which genes these loci correspond to. Genetics could soon be involved in drug development, and gene therapy would enhance clinical decision making.

Presentation

Osteoporosis is considered a "silent disease," and is often missed in elderly individuals. Osteoporosis screening[22] is therefore essential and recommended for women 65 years and older and women younger than 65 who are postmenopausal with risk factors. Screening includes yearly dual energy x-ray absorptiometry scans to measure BMD at the hip and lumbar spine. The National Osteoporosis Foundation guidelines recommend BMD measurement for women aged 65 and older and men aged 70 and older, regardless of risk factors. If risk factors are present, screening is recommended for younger postmenopausal women, women in menopausal transition, and men aged 50 to 59.[23]

Fragility fracture refers to a break in the bone in a low-impact trauma setting that would typically not cause a fracture. As patients age, studies have found that osteoporotic women suffer more than 3 times more nonvertebral fractures than those with normal BMD.[24] Most nonvertebral fractures are related to falls, whereas most vertebral compression fractures occur in the absence of a fall.[25] Previous studies suggest that a fragility fracture occurs with increased load on the spine, and can even occur during trivial events such as sneezing or lying in bed.[26] The most common locations of vertebral fractures are at the T12 and L2 segments, both which include transitions from rigid thoracic vertebrae to mobile lumbar vertebrae.

The classic description of a vertebral fragility fracture is an osteoporotic individual experiencing severe back pain while bending forward. Nevertheless, in an aging athlete, compression fracture can present similar to a muscle strain. This variation in presentation of spinal compression fractures can result in inaccuracy. Vertebral fractures are often the most common complication but remain undiagnosed because they are mostly asymptomatic.[13,27]

Often, the only symptom of vertebral compression fracture is low back pain. However, due to prolonged activity, there are increased risks of deep vein thrombosis and pulmonary embolism. Multiple vertebral fractures can cause fatigued muscles and pain, causing difficulty in maintaining posture. Continued loss of vertebral body height can eventually result in deformities such as thoracic kyphosis and lumbar lordosis, impairing gait and balance. In severe cases, vertebral fractures can impair pulmonary function and cause early satiety, weight loss, and morbidity and mortality.[28,29]

Assessment for Fracture Risk

One of the most commonly used algorithms to assess BMD and its risk factors for fracture risk is FRAX[30] or a variation called DeFRA,[31] which uses continuous variables and is considered to be more detailed. The risk factors for the World Health Organization Fracture Risk Assessment Model include age, gender, body mass index, prior osteoporotic fracture, femoral neck BMD, rheumatoid arthritis, secondary causes of osteoporosis, parental history of hip fracture, current smoking, alcohol intake, and oral glucocorticoids.[30,32]

Osteoporosis Prevention and Nonpharmacologic Management

Lifestyle changes and exercise

Patients can regain significant bone health by making lifestyle changes, including increasing physical activity and reducing smoking and drinking. Two types of exercise remain most beneficial for osteoporosis: (1) weight-bearing aerobic exercises, such as walking, stair climbing, tai chi, and dancing; and (2) strength training/resistance exercises like free weights. Low weight-bearing exercises, which include stair stepping machines and elliptical training machines are alternatives for those who cannot perform high-impact exercises. Studies also show that walking and cycling are not as beneficial, and clinicians theorize that physical activity must induce some sort of mechanical stress to help stimulate bone mass.[33,34] Most studies have analyzed current athletes rather than former athletes. However, several studies have found that lumbar spine BMD was significantly higher in athletes who competed in long jumping, pole vaulting, and triple jump compared with endurance runners, with the highest BMD in rugby players.[35,36]

Although there are limited studies, the exercise most effective for osteoporosis at the spine is multicomponent training. Gravitational stress is another element that is beneficial in exercise, with those who played tennis having a higher BMD than the counterparts who swam.[37]

Peak bone mass has shown to be associated with decreased fracture risk even if resistance training is not maintained.[38] Nevertheless, this does not imply working out at a young age ensures optimal BMD at an older age; people who exercise have a higher BMD than those that do not. Other benefits of exercise include decreased dementia, diabetes, depression, anxiety, fatigue, cardiac death, and ischemic heart disease.

Nutrition

Diets high in calcium and vitamin D are essential to help maintain bone mass.[39] The Food and Nutrition Board recommends that men older than 70 and postmenopausal women consume 800 IU (200g) of vitamin D each day. Health care providers may supplement further to reduce the risk of osteoporosis.[39,40] Adequate sources of calcium include green vegetables, milk, and other dairy products, such as yogurt and hard cheese.[41]

Fall prevention

The most common cause of fractures is osteoporosis. Osteoporosis prevention must incorporate falling prevention.[42] Fall prevention has shown to help reduce osteoporosis-related morbidity.[43] Patients can reduce fall risk by fall-proofing the house and modifying patients' activities.[42] For example, patients can

a. Remove loose rugs, and include adequate lighting in all areas inside and around the house
b. Avoid walking on slippery surfaces
c. Review drug regimen to avoid causing an imbalance

Pharmacologic management

Bisphosphonates are first-line medications for osteoporosis management and it is necessary to reassess after three to 5 years for fracture risk.[44] Alternative treatments include Denosumab and Teriparatide/Abaloparatide (Parathyroid hormone (PTH) and PTH-related protein analogs). Patients on Denosumab monotherapy can be reassessed after 5 to 10 years. PTH analogs are considered in severe or multiple vertebral fractures for up to 2 years. Newer medications like anabolic steroids (Romosozumab) have shown to be effective in severe osteoporosis, but are only used after failed treatments.

DEGENERATIVE DISK DISEASE
Overview

Degenerative disk disease (DDD) refers to degeneration of the intervertebral disk characterized by disk dehydration, annular tear, and loss of disk height.[45] Intervertebral disks are cartilaginous structures that lie between vertebral bodies connecting them. They consist of 2 rings, annulus fibrosis, a thick outer ring of fibrous cartilage, and the nucleus pulposus, a gelatinous core.[46,47] Disruption of these disks can cause herniation of the nucleus pulposus. DDD specifically refers to disk degeneration that causes pain and/or neurologic symptoms.

This is a common phenomenon in elderly individuals, as more than 90% of adults by the age of 60 will show a small amount of disk degeneration.[46] A high number of elite athletes had significant spinal degeneration at the 2016 Olympics.[48] Almost 52% showed severe spinal disease, with the highest level of degeneration indicating potential association with cyclic overloading speeding up cell death within cells. The most frequent site is the thoracolumbar junction due to flexion, extension, and rotation loads that increase disk strain and stress. Football, wrestling, hockey, dance, gymnastics, tennis, and golf are individual sports in which this injury mechanism commonly occurs, whereas runners were not affected by DDD.

Risk Factors

a. Aging and genetics (most important)
b. Excessive strain on the disk, such as sports, heavy lifting, and labor-intensive jobs; type of sport and intensity has shown acceleration of disk degeneration (75% of elite gymnasts show DDD)
c. Sedentary lifestyle: prolonged sitting can strain the back and cause excessive gravitational load on the spine
d. Trauma on the disk: surgery or fracture slowing blood supply
e. Smoking

Presentation

The patient's history, physical examination, and events before presentation of symptoms should be recounted. MRI should not be ordered unless red flags, such as cauda equina, infection, suspected tumor, or trauma (fall, collision), are present. Radiation of back pain associated with disk disease is thought to be due to the compression of nerve roots in the spinal canal from either disk herniation or hypertrophy of the degenerative tissues. The nucleus pulposus is resorbed over time. Other times, the ligamentum flavum and the facet joints can compromise the surrounding nerve roots.[46] Acute sciatica often remains undiagnosed due to its increased variation in its presentation: people report only 8% acute sciatica after heavy lifting or physical trauma.[49]

Diagnosis

The initial study of choice is an upright radiograph to rule out deformity, fractures, and neoplastic causes of low back pain. MRI is the more sensitive imaging modality to assess disk disease, like disk space narrowing, decreased signal intensity in the disk, and vertebral endplate changes. T2-weighted MRI can be used to assess for any compression of neurologic structures.

Management

Initial management includes physical therapy and the use of nonsteroidal anti-inflammatory drugs or epidural infections. Epidural injections may provide short-term relief but long-term relief has not been shown.[50,51] The nonconservative approach does not work for many people and discectomy is typically offered. According to the SPORT trial, patients electing for surgery had better outcomes both at 3 months and 4 years.[52] Data are not available regarding elderly athletes, but younger athletes return 5 months after operation. Postoperative rehabilitation with intensive exercise programs showed considerable improvement and return to function than mild intensity programs. High-intensity programs were not associated with reherniation or reoperation. It is important to keep in mind that surgery is not a cure-all for disk degeneration and will not reverse the damage. Weight loss, an exercise program, and a healthy diet are essential, and positive changes in lifestyle have shown significant improvement in symptoms.[53] Mature athletes must also be cognizant of their limitations. They might have to alter exercise and activity levels with the help of physical therapy to reduce pain in the lower back and stress on the disk.

SPINAL STENOSIS
Overview

Spinal stenosis is characterized as compression of the nerve roots and spinal cord, causing symptoms including pain, numbness, or weakness. There are 3 main mechanisms that spinal stenosis can affect the aging spine. First, narrowing of the central canal, which contains the spinal cord, can cause reduction of blood supply and compression of neural structures. Second, compression of the neural foramen, opening where nerve roots exit the spinal cord, can occur. Finally, the lateral recess in the lumbar spine, where the nerve root enters before it exits the neural foramen, can be compressed by facet joint hypertrophy.[54]

The prevalence of spinal stenosis increases by age and is predicted to be 19.4% for people aged 60 to 69.[55] Lumbar spinal surgery (LSS) remains the most common reason for the elderly to undergo spinal surgery and in 2009, the hospital costs for LSS was $1.6 billion.[56]

There are limited studies analyzing the prevalence of spinal stenosis in athletes. As opposed to solely being caused by a degenerative process, lumbar stenosis in athletes can be caused by scoliosis, spondylolisthesis, or lumbar disk herniation. Athletes in contact sports, like football players, can experience neuropraxia with a severe hyperextension injury. This cohort was found to have an increased prevalence of cervical spine stenosis. Meanwhile, masters athletes do not typically participate in contact sports[57]; yet, weight-lifting and swimming competitions have been shown to involve extensive extension forces that could potentially cause symptomatic stenosis seen in contact sports.

Presentation

Pain in spinal stenosis often originates as lumbar pain that progressively worsens and causes numbness. Neurogenic claudication remains the most common symptom and can lead to positional pain and weakness that is worse while walking, but improves as one bends forward or sits. Symptoms are often more acute as the disease progresses.

Diagnosis

Lumbar MRI is the gold standard to visualize the greatest change associated with spinal stenosis. T1-weighted and T2-weighted images are obtained in sagittal and transverse planes. Radiographs may be useful to see degenerative changes; computed tomography (CT) scans help assess bone condition and diagnose osteoporosis. Other diagnostic evaluations to rule in or out other differentials include ankle brachial index, laboratory tests such as HbA1c, C-reactive protein, complete blood count, and further neurology workup if there is suspicion of polyneuropathy.

Management

According to Johnsson and colleagues,[58] 70% of patients remain stable for a 4-year period, 15% improve, and 15% become worse. Pharmacologic management includes muscle relaxants and painkillers as required, but care must be taken when managing pain in elderly individuals. Opioids, such as gabapentin, must be balanced with cognitive side effects, but they have therapeutic effects associated with neurologic damage. Nonsteroidal anti-inflammatory drugs (NSAIDs) and acetaminophen have renal and hepatic side effects, respectively, and can predispose to gastric ulcers, so must be used with caution. Physiotherapy, including massage, exercises, and manipulation, pain management, and lifestyle modification are essential to recovery. Although existing reports suggest that exercise may lead to exacerbation of symptoms, exercise is important in conditioning and strengthening the back or lumbar muscles, avoiding weakening or further impairment. No evidence exists to suggest that one type of therapy is superior. Wearing braces such as corsets has shown no improvement.[59] Stationary bikes have been well tolerated by athletes as they prepare to return from injury.

Epidural injections have been shown to reduce inflammation and provide pain relief. Epidural injections with anesthetic properties and steroids have shown no benefit compared with the anesthetic alone.[60,61] The procedure itself can be difficult to perform in adults with degenerative changes. In terms of long-term pain relief and function, epidural injections do not have an effect.[62,63]

Surgery is the ultimate option for management in patients who have severe limitations of function. In patients older than 65 who are undergoing spine surgery, lumbar spinal stenosis is the most common preoperative diagnosis.[64] There are many procedural techniques and minimal guidelines on which treatment to use. Without spondylolisthesis, laminectomy and fusion were found to be superior to nonoperative approaches.[65] Decompression with fusion leads to high intraoperative blood loss and does not improve postoperative complications compared with decompression alone.[66] Recently, minimally invasive decompression procedures or surgeries have become more common and studies demonstrate an association with higher patient satisfaction with similar complication rates.[67] Another minimally invasive technique that uses interspinous processes can reduce operative time, but has not shown much improvement to current standard, and in fact, has been associated with higher rates of reoperation.[68,69]

Prevention

Currently, athletes are cross-training and strengthening their muscles to maintain balance between lower extremity and trunk flexors and extensors. This can reduce the hyperextension loads that exacerbate the symptoms of lumbar stenosis. For example, weight lifters focus on full-body conditioning, flexibility, aerobic conditioning, speed, and cross-training. Although running solely does not predispose to lumbar stenosis, runners with risk factors or prior history can focus on improving flexibility and strengthening the abdominal and spinal stabilizing musculature.

Facet Joint Arthritis

Facet joint pain is present between 15% and 52% of the average population, with an increased percentage in elderly athletes due to degenerative arthritis.[70,71] Each vertebra is composed of a 3-joint complex that comprises 2 paired facet joints and the intervertebral disk.[72] Each joint is composed of cartilage and synovial fluid to maintain mobility of joints. Facet joint (FJ) arthritis is a degenerative change between joints that can break down cartilage and form bone spurs. This is typically caused by aging, but can be heightened by repetitive extension, flexion, and torsion of the lumbar spine.[73] There is a significant association with age, as 89% of people aged 65 and older are noted to have FJ arthritis on CT imaging.[74] However, athletes can accelerate the degeneration process by using more repetitive extension motions, which is often seen in golfers, throwers, or gymnasts.

Presentation

The symptoms of FJ arthritis can range from being asymptomatic to pseudo-radicular lumbar pain. Although referral patterns of FJ are varied, the pain can be referred distally to the lower limbs causing a pseudo-radicular syndrome. The pain typically ends above the knee, but extends to the feet if complicated by osteophytes. Moreover, FJ arthritis can have claudication-type sensations, with pain worsening in the mornings and during periods of inactivity. The pain can be elicited at times during lumbar extension or FJ palpation.

Diagnosis

After eliminating disk herniation, spinal stenosis, and other immediate neurologic causes, FJ osteoarthritis can be higher on the differential. It is considered a rule-out diagnosis, as it does not produce consistent, specific symptoms. There are no physical examination maneuvers that can diagnose FJ arthritis. CT is the most sensitive technique, although MRI can be used to visualize surrounding soft tissues. Some studies have shown that MRI and other imaging modalities have not been reliable in diagnosing FJ osteoarthritis.[75,76] The most common features found on imaging include narrowing of the facet joint space, subarticular bone erosion, subchondral cyst, and osteophyte formation.[72] Other invasive procedures like facet blocks have been used to identify and confirm the diagnosis, but can be associated with false positive rates.[77,78]

Management

Conservative management is considered first-line treatment in many cases. It is important to properly teach the patient about daily posture and exercise. Physical therapy can similarly be useful to restore posture and strengthen abdominal and neck flexor muscles to balance the extensors. Multimodal pain management consisting of NSAIDs, muscle relaxants, and acetaminophen can be used during acute flares.

There are more invasive techniques like ultrasound-guided facet blocks, which demonstrate 82% effectiveness for approximately 6 months.[79] Steroid injections, however, have inconsistent data, suggesting they might be less beneficial in the management of chronic lower back pain.[77,80] Neurolysis, denervation of nerve fibers resulting in regeneration, is another technique reporting promising results. Neurolysis does not provide a permanent solution, but studies indicate that almost 60% of patients can expect 90% of pain reduction and 87% can expect 60% reduction lasting 12 months.[81] No guidelines exist for surgical management. If complicated by spondylolisthesis or severe pain, lumbar decompressive laminectomy can provide relief occasionally.[82]

Spondylolysis/Spondylolisthesis

Spondylolysis is a defect of the pars interarticularis, which can be induced by trauma, stress fracture, or recurrent microtrauma. Spondylolisthesis refers to the slipping of a vertebral body with respect to the adjacent body.[83] The most common sites of injury are L5-S1 vertebrae followed by L4-L5. The main cause of spondylolisthesis is degenerative but athletes are at a higher risk. It is postulated that there could be microtrauma caused by repetitive lumbar extension from various activities like gymnastics, football, and wrestling. It is estimated that spondylolisthesis causes 70% to 80% of low back pain in adolescent athletes.[84] Previous studies estimate that the prevalence of spondylolysis in wrestlers and weight lifters is 30% and 23%, respectively, compared with 6% to 18% of the US population.[83,85,86] Other risk factors for spondylolisthesis include anatomic variations such as spina bifida or scoliosis.

Presentation

Spondylolisthesis has an asymptomatic nature and often recognized incidentally. The pain is usually exacerbating with flexion and extension at the site of slippage. Direct pressure may also cause pain. Lying supine diminishes the pain by opening up the spinal canal and relieving pressure on the bony elements. A radiculopathy component can be identified, as nerve roots can be compressed, leading to narrowing of the nerve.

Diagnosis

Radiography is necessary for initial management and diagnosis of spondylolisthesis. It is possible to see abnormal alignment of the vertebral body or a pars defect, which can indicate ischemic spondylolisthesis. CT scan has the highest sensitivity and specificity. MRI can identify small tissues, but does not aid in visualization of the pars defect.

Management

Conservative management is considered first-line treatment. Orthoses are external devices that are flexible or rigid. There are 2 main types: thoracolumbosacral and lumbosacral orthoses. Flexible versions are used to decrease activity of paraspinal muscles and increase abdominal pressure. Rigid orthoses are effective in limited sagittal plane motion, but have limited control over rotation and lateral bending. Some studies have demonstrated little to no immobilization effect from wearing orthoses.

North American Spine Society spondylolisthesis guidelines suggest that surgical decompression may be considered for patients with low-grade degenerative spondylolisthesis that is refractory to conservative management. Many studies have also shown that fusion may have improved long-term outcomes compared with surgical decompression alone, but with increased surgical morbidity.

SUMMARY

Aging athletes continue to increase in number, and it is important to recognize the increased spine care risk this cohort faces, as well as treatment options to safely return these athletes back to competition. It is important to recognize the warning signs and adjust the workout before injury in these athletes. Patient education to prevent reinjury is crucial to maintain a healthy and active lifestyle.

DISCLOSURE

The authors have nothing to disclose.

REFERENCES

1. Fatoye F, Gebrye T, Odeyemi I. Real-world incidence and prevalence of low back pain using routinely collected data. Rheumatol Int 2019;39(4):619–26.
2. Hughes VA, Frontera WR, Roubenoff R, et al. Longitudinal changes in body composition in older men and women: role of body weight change and physical activity. Am J Clin Nutr 2002;76(2):473–81.
3. Melov S, Shoffner JM, Kaufman A, et al. Marked increase in the number and variety of mitochondrial DNA rearrangements in aging human skeletal muscle. Nucleic Acids Res 1995;23(20):4122–6.
4. Lamberts SW, van den Beld AW, van der Lely AJ. The endocrinology of aging. Science 1997;278(5337):419–24.
5. Oxidative Stress, Caloric Restriction, and Aging | Ovid. Available at: https://oce.ovid.com/article/00007529-199607050-00002. Accessed July 29, 2020.
6. Pouresmaeili F, Kamalidehghan B, Kamarehei M, et al. A comprehensive overview on osteoporosis and its risk factors. Ther Clin Risk Manag 2018;14:2029–49.
7. World Health Organization. WHO scientific group on the assessment of osteoporosis at the primary health care level: summary meeting report. Brussels, Belgium; May 5–7, 2004. Published online 2007.
8. Wright N, et al. Abstract 1079. Presented at: American Society of Bone and Mineral Research Annual Meeting; September 20–23, 2019; Orlando.
9. Burge R, Dawson-Hughes B, Solomon DH, et al. Incidence and economic burden of osteoporosis-related fractures in the United States, 2005-2025. J Bone Miner Res 2007;22(3):465–75.
10. Lane NE. Epidemiology, etiology, and diagnosis of osteoporosis. Am J Obstet Gynecol 2006;194(2):S3–11.
11. Waugh EJ, Lam M-A, Hawker GA, et al. Risk factors for low bone mass in healthy 40–60 year old women: a systematic review of the literature. Osteoporos Int 2008; 20(1):1.

12. Rosen CJ. The epidemiology and pathogenesis of osteoporosis. In: Feingold KR, Anawalt B, Boyce A, et al., eds Endotext. MDText.com, Inc. 2000. Available at: http://www.ncbi.nlm.nih.gov/books/NBK279134/. Accessed July 9, 2020.

13. Wright NC, Looker AC, Saag KG, et al. The recent prevalence of osteoporosis and low bone mass in the United States based on bone mineral density at the femoral neck or lumbar spine. J Bone Miner Res 2014;29(11):2520–6.

14. Looker AC, Borrud LG, Dawson-Hughes B, et al. Osteoporosis or low bone mass at the femur neck or lumbar spine in older adults: United States, 2005-2008. NCHS Data Brief 2012;(93):1–8.

15. Looker AC, Melton LJ, Harris TB, et al. Prevalence and trends in low femur bone density among older US adults: NHANES 2005-2006 compared with NHANES III. J Bone Miner Res 2010;25(1):64–71.

16. Benedetti MG, Furlini G, Zati A, et al. The effectiveness of physical exercise on bone density in osteoporotic patients. Biomed Res Int 2018. https://doi.org/10.1155/2018/4840531.

17. Al-Bashaireh AM, Haddad LG, Weaver M, et al. The effect of tobacco smoking on bone mass: an overview of pathophysiologic mechanisms. J Osteoporos 2018. https://doi.org/10.1155/2018/1206235.

18. Sahni S, Mangano KM, McLean RR, et al. Dietary approaches for bone health: lessons from the Framingham Osteoporosis Study. Curr Osteoporos Rep 2015; 13(4):245–55.

19. Sahni S, Mangano KM, Kiel DP, et al. Dairy intake is protective against bone loss in older vitamin D supplement users: the Framingham Study123. J Nutr 2017; 147(4):645–52.

20. Al Anouti F, Taha Z, Shamim S, et al. An insight into the paradigms of osteoporosis: from genetics to biomechanics. Bone Rep 2019;11:100216.

21. Morris JA, Kemp JP, Youlten SE, et al. An atlas of genetic influences on osteoporosis in humans and mice. Nat Genet 2019;51(2):258–66.

22. Osteoporosis to prevent fractures: screening | healthy people. Available at: https://www.healthypeople.gov/2020/tools-resources/evidence-based-resource/osteoporosis-to-prevent-fractures-screening. Accessed July 15, 2020.

23. Bone density test, osteoporosis screening & T-score Interpretation. National Osteoporosis Foundation. Available at: https://www.nof.org/patients/diagnosis-information/bone-density-examtesting/. Accessed July 15, 2020.

24. Siris ES, Chen Y-T, Abbott TA, et al. Bone mineral density thresholds for pharmacological intervention to prevent fractures. Arch Intern Med 2004;164(10): 1108–12.

25. Cummings SR, Nevitt MC. Non-skeletal determinants of fractures: the potential importance of the mechanics of falls. Study of Osteoporotic Fractures Research Group. Osteoporos Int 1994;4(Suppl 1):67–70.

26. Bostrom MP, Lane JM. Future directions. Augmentation of osteoporotic vertebral bodies. Spine 1997;22(24 Suppl):38S–42S.

27. Ensrud KE. Epidemiology of fracture risk with advancing age. J Gerontol A Biol Sci Med Sci 2013;68(10):1236–42.

28. Vaccaro AR, Kim DH, Brodke DS, et al. Diagnosis and management of thoracolumbar spine fractures. Instr Course Lect 2004;53:359–73.

29. Lindsay R, Burge RT, Strauss DM. One year outcomes and costs following a vertebral fracture. Osteoporos Int 2005;16(1):78–85.

30. Available at: https://www.sheffield.ac.uk/FRAX/tool.aspx?country=9. Accessed July 9, 2020.

31. DeFRA - Home. Available at: https://defra-osteoporosi.it/. Accessed July 15, 2020.
32. Kanis JA, on behalf of the World Health Organization Scientific Group. Assessment of osteoporosis at the primary health care level. Technical Report. South Yorkshire, England: United Kingdom: World Health Organization Collaborating Center for Metabolic Bone Diseases. University of Sheffield; 2007.
33. Kelley GA, Kelley KS, Kohrt WM. Effects of ground and joint reaction force exercise on lumbar spine and femoral neck bone mineral density in postmenopausal women: a meta-analysis of randomized controlled trials. BMC Musculoskelet Disord 2012;13(1):177.
34. Hingorjo MR, Zehra S, Saleem S, et al. Serum interleukin-15 and its relationship with adiposity indices before and after short-term endurance exercise | Hingorjo | Pakistan Journal of Medical Sciences Old Website. Available at: http://pjms.com.pk/index.php/pjms/article/view/15516. Accessed July 9, 2020.
35. Schmitt H, Friebe C, Schneider S, et al. Bone mineral density and degenerative changes of the lumbar spine in former elite athletes. Int J Sports Med 2005; 26(6):457–63.
36. Nevill AM, Holder RL, Stewart AD. Do sporting activities convey benefits to bone mass throughout the skeleton? J Sports Sci 2004;22(7):645–50.
37. Jacobson PC, Beaver W, Grubb SA, et al. Bone density in women: college athletes and older athletic women. J Orthop Res 1984;2(4):328–32.
38. The aging spine in sports- ClinicalKey. Available at: https://www.clinicalkey.com/#!/content/playContent/1-s2.0-S027859191200018X?scrollTo=%23hl0000073. Accessed July 17, 2020.
39. Nuti R, Brandi ML, Checchia G, et al. Guidelines for the management of osteoporosis and fragility fractures. Intern Emerg Med 2019;14(1):85.
40. Khazai N, Judd SE, Tangpricha V. Calcium and vitamin D: skeletal and extraskeletal health. Curr Rheumatol Rep 2008;10(2):110–7.
41. Cormick G, Belizán JM. Calcium intake and health. Nutrients 2019;11(7). https://doi.org/10.3390/nu11071606.
42. Cosman F, de Beur SJ, LeBoff MS, et al. Clinician's guide to prevention and treatment of osteoporosis. Osteoporos Int 2014;25(10):2359–81.
43. Preventing falls and related fractures | NIH Osteoporosis and Related Bone Diseases National Resource Center. Available at: https://www.bones.nih.gov/health-info/bone/osteoporosis/fracture/preventing-falls-and-related-fractures. Accessed July 15, 2020.
44. Shoback D, Rosen CJ, Black DM, et al. Pharmacological management of osteoporosis in postmenopausal women: an Endocrine Society guideline update. J Clin Endocrinol Metab 2020;105(3):587–94.
45. Trainor TJ, Trainor MA. Etiology of low back pain in athletes. Curr Sports Med Rep 2004;3(1):41–6.
46. Donnally CJ III, Hanna A, Varacallo M. Lumbar degenerative disk disease. In: StatPearls. Treasure Island (FL): StatPearls Publishing; 2020. Available at: http://www.ncbi.nlm.nih.gov/books/NBK448134/. Accessed July 17, 2020.
47. Hicks GE, Morone N, Weiner DK. Degenerative lumbar disc and facet disease in older adults. Spine (Phila Pa 1976) 2009;34(12):1301–6.
48. Evaluation of spine MRIs in athletes participating in the Rio de Janeiro 2016 Summer Olympic Games | BMJ Open Sport & Exercise Medicine. Available at: https://bmjopensem.bmj.com/content/4/1/e000335. Accessed July 17, 2020.
49. Yao Q, Wang S, Shin J-H, et al. Lumbar facet joint motion in patients with degenerative spondylolisthesis. J Spinal Disord Tech 2013;26(1):E19–27.

50. Choi HJ, Hahn S, Kim CH, et al. Epidural steroid injection therapy for low back pain: a meta-analysis. Int J Technol Assess Health Care 2013;29(3):244–53.

51. Buttermann GR. The effect of spinal steroid injections for degenerative disc disease. Spine J 2004;4(5):495–505.

52. Weinstein JN, Tosteson TD, Lurie JD, et al. Surgical vs nonoperative treatment for lumbar disk herniation: The Spine Patient Outcomes Research Trial (SPORT): a randomized trial. JAMA 2006;296(20):2441–50.

53. Malham GM, Parker RM, Blecher CM, et al. Choice of approach does not affect clinical and radiologic outcomes: a comparative cohort of patients having anterior lumbar interbody fusion and patients having lateral lumbar interbody fusion at 24 months. Glob Spine J 2016;6(5):472–81.

54. Raja A, Hoang S, Viswanath O, et al. Spinal stenosis. In: StatPearls. Treasure Island (FL): StatPearls Publishing; 2020. Available at: http://www.ncbi.nlm.nih.gov/books/NBK441989/. Accessed July 29, 2020.

55. Wu A-M, Zou F, Cao Y, et al. Lumbar spinal stenosis: an update on the epidemiology, diagnosis and treatment. AME Med J 2017;2(5). Available at: http://amj.amegroups.com/article/view/3837. Accessed July 18, 2020.

56. Deyo RA, Mirza SK, Martin BI, et al. Trends, major medical complications, and charges associated with surgery for lumbar spinal stenosis in older adults. JAMA 2010;303(13):1259–65.

57. Mayer JE, Cho SK, Qureshi SA, et al. Cervical spine injury in athletes. Curr Orthop Pract 2012;23(3):181–7.

58. Johnsson KE, Rosén I, Udén A. The natural course of lumbar spinal stenosis. Clin Orthop Relat Res 1992;279:82–6.

59. Macedo LG, Hum A, Kuleba L, et al. Physical therapy interventions for degenerative lumbar spinal stenosis: a systematic review. Phys Ther 2013;93(12):1646–60.

60. Friedly JL, Comstock BA, Turner JA, et al. A randomized trial of epidural glucocorticoid injections for spinal stenosis. N Engl J Med 2014;371(1):11–21.

61. Fukusaki M, Kobayashi I, Hara T, et al. Symptoms of spinal stenosis do not improve after epidural steroid injection. Clin J Pain 1998;14(2):148–51.

62. Jordan SE. Assessment: use of epidural steroid injections to treat radicular lumbosacral pain: report of the Therapeutics and Technology Assessment Subcommittee of the American Academy of Neurology. Neurology 2007;69(11):1191 [author reply: 1191–2].

63. Chou R, Hashimoto R, Friedly J, et al. Epidural corticosteroid injections for radiculopathy and spinal stenosis: a systematic review and meta-analysis. Ann Intern Med 2015;163(5):373–81.

64. Munakomi S, Foris LA, Varacallo M. Spinal stenosis and neurogenic claudication. In: StatPearls. Treasure Island (FL): StatPearls Publishing; 2020. Available at: http://www.ncbi.nlm.nih.gov/books/NBK430872/. Accessed July 29, 2020.

65. Ghogawala Z, Resnick DK, Glassman SD, et al. Randomized controlled trials for degenerative lumbar spondylolisthesis: which patients benefit from lumbar fusion? J Neurosurg Spine 2017;26(2):260–6.

66. Machado GC, Ferreira PH, Harris IA, et al. Effectiveness of surgery for lumbar spinal stenosis: a systematic review and meta-analysis. PLoS One 2015;10(3). https://doi.org/10.1371/journal.pone.0122800.

67. Phan K, Mobbs RJ. Minimally invasive versus open laminectomy for lumbar stenosis: a systematic review and meta-analysis. Spine 2016;41(2):E91–100.

68. X-stop versus decompressive surgery for lumbar neurogenic intermittent claudication: randomized controlled trial with 2-year follow-up - PubMed. Available at: https://pubmed.ncbi.nlm.nih.gov/23403549/. Accessed July 29, 2020.

69. Moojen WA, Arts MP, Jacobs WCH, et al. Interspinous process device versus standard conventional surgical decompression for lumbar spinal stenosis: randomized controlled trial. BMJ 2013;347:f6415.

70. Gadia A, Shah K, Nene A. Outcomes of various treatment modalities for lumbar spinal ailments in elite athletes: a literature review. Asian Spine J 2018;12(4): 754–64.

71. Manchikanti L, Singh V, Pampati V, et al. Evaluation of the relative contributions of various structures in chronic low back pain. Pain Physician 2001;4(4):308–16.

72. Gellhorn AC, Katz JN, Suri P. Osteoarthritis of the spine: the facet joints. Nat Rev Rheumatol 2013;9(4):216–24.

73. Watkins RG, Dillin WH. Lumbar spine injury in the athlete. Clin Sports Med 1990; 9(2):419–48.

74. Suri P, Miyakoshi A, Hunter DJ, et al. Does lumbar spinal degeneration begin with the anterior structures? A study of the observed epidemiology in a community-based population. BMC Musculoskelet Disord 2011;12:202.

75. Kjaer P, Leboeuf-Yde C, Korsholm L, et al. Magnetic resonance imaging and low back pain in adults: a diagnostic imaging study of 40-year-old men and women. Spine 2005;30(10):1173–80.

76. Hechelhammer L, Pfirrmann CWA, Zanetti M, et al. Imaging findings predicting the outcome of cervical facet joint blocks. Eur Radiol 2007;17(4):959–64.

77. Cohen SP, Raja SN. Pathogenesis, diagnosis, and treatment of lumbar zygapophysial (facet) joint pain. Anesthesiology 2007;106(3):591–614.

78. van Kleef M, Vanelderen P, Cohen SP, et al. 12. Pain originating from the lumbar facet joints. Pain Pract 2010;10(5):459–69.

79. Manchikanti L, Malla Y, Wargo BW, et al. Complications of fluoroscopically directed facet joint nerve blocks: a prospective evaluation of 7,500 episodes with 43,000 nerve blocks. Pain Physician 2012;15(2):E143–50.

80. Lilius G, Laasonen EM, Myllynen P, et al. Lumbar facet joint syndrome. A randomised clinical trial. J Bone Joint Surg Br 1989;71(4):681–4.

81. Dreyfuss P, Halbrook B, Pauza K, et al. Efficacy and validity of radiofrequency neurotomy for chronic lumbar zygapophysial joint pain. Spine 2000;25(10): 1270–7.

82. Perolat R, Kastler A, Nicot B, et al. Facet joint syndrome: from diagnosis to interventional management. Insights Imaging 2018;9(5):773–89.

83. Tenny S, Gillis CC. Spondylolisthesis. In: StatPearls. Treasure Island (FL): StatPearls Publishing; 2020. Available at: http://www.ncbi.nlm.nih.gov/books/NBK430767/. Accessed July 29, 2020.

84. Standaert CJ, Herring SA. Spondylolysis: a critical review. Br J Sports Med 2000; 34(6):415–22.

85. Rossi F, Dragoni S. Lumbar spondylolysis: occurrence in competitive athletes. Updated achievements in a series of 390 cases. J Sports Med Phys Fitness 1990;30(4):450–2.

86. Soler T, Calderón C. The prevalence of spondylolysis in the Spanish elite athlete. Am J Sports Med 2000;28(1):57–62.